Towards a European
art therapy

Towards a European art therapy

Creating a profession

Diane Waller

Open University Press
Buckingham · Philadelphia

Open University Press
Celtic Court
22 Ballmoor
Buckingham
MK18 1XW

email: enquiries@openup.co.uk
world wide web: http://www.openup.co.uk

and
325 Chestnut Street
Philadelphia, PA 19106, USA

First Published 1998

Copyright © Diane Waller 1998

All rights reserved. Except for the quotation of short passages for the purpose of criticism and review, no part of this publication may be reproduced, stored in a retrieval system, or transmitted, in any form or by any means, electronic, mechanical, photocopying, recording or otherwise, without the prior written permission of the publisher or a licence from the Copyright Licensing Agency Limited. Details of such licences (for reprographic reproduction) may be obtained from the Copyright Licensing Agency Ltd of 90 Tottenham Court Road, London W1P 9HE.

A catalogue record of this book is available from the British Library

ISBN 0 335 19448 6 (pbk)   0 335 19449 4 (hbk)

Library of Congress Cataloging-in-Publication Data
Waller. Diane, 1943–
    Towards a European art therapy: creating a profession/Diane Waller.
      p. cm.
    Includes bibliographical references and index.
    ISBN 0–335–19449–4 (hbk). – ISBN 0–335–19448–6 (pbk.)
    1. Art therapy–Europe. 2. Psychotherapy–Europe. I. Title.
RC489.A7W367 1998
615.8'5156'094–dc21   98–5419
                                                                                    CIP

Typeset by Graphicraft Limited, Hong Kong
Printed in Great Britain by St Edmundsbury Press Ltd,
Bury St Edmunds, Suffolk

In loving memory of my husband Dan Lumley, who died on 4 July 1998, and who contributed so much to this book and to all my previous work.

Contents

Acknowledgements and notes on contributors	ix
1 Introduction: the need for a European perspective	1
Part I Case studies	7
2 Art therapy in Ireland *Deirdre Horgan*	9
3 Art therapy in Switzerland *Jacques Stitelmann*	29
Part II The profession	45
4 Definitions, limits and boundaries	47
5 Ownership and regulation	63
6 Social and cultural contexts	76
Part III Training and development	97
7 Training	99
8 Professional development	129
Part IV Conclusion	141
9 Present and future	143
Bibliography	148
Useful contacts	159
Index	162

Acknowledgements and notes on contributors

I would like to thank most sincerely those people who have contributed to the development of this book, either by preparing for me very succinct papers or by gathering information about the art therapy profession in their own country, or both. They are listed below and their contributions are drawn upon frequently in the text. Most of these contributors are correspondents for the International Networking Group of Art Therapists, founded by Bobbi Stoll when she was President of the American Art Therapists Association to whom grateful thanks for this initiative. I hope everyone will feel justice has been done to their efforts. Others to be thanked are: the Central Research Committee of the University of London for a grant towards the research for this book; Val Huet and Susan Chalkley for help with French translation; Pat Capocci for helping to type it; the Council for Professions Supplementary to Medicine (CPSM) for affording me so many opportunities to get familiar with European Directives; Joan Malherbe and Jacinta Evans of Open University Press for their support. I also hope that those people who didn't know about the planned book, (or whom I didn't know about) who would like to send me information about their or others' activities will do so, and perhaps there can be a Volume 2 or second edition at a later date.

Special thanks to those who made the book possible and who have been quoted extensively:

x   *Acknowledgements and notes on contributors*

Karin Dannecker: Lecturer in art therapy at the Hochschule der Kunst, Berlin and Senior Art Therapist at the Schlosspark Klinic in Berlin. Currently engaged in a collaborative outcome research project with Diane Waller.
Mimma Della Cagnoletta: Director of training at Art Therapy Italiana, Bologna and former President of ATI. Lives and works privately as an art therapist in Milan.
Deirdre Horgan: Art therapist working in adult and child psychiatry in Ireland. Lecturer in art therapy to several multiprofessional groups and engaged in the professional development of arts therapy through the Irish Association.
Wolfgang Mastnak: Until recently Head of Arts Therapies at the University Mozarteum, Salzburg. Visiting lecturer to universities in Prague, Bratislava, Cologne and Munich, and pioneer of integrative arts therapy in Austria.
Jacques Stitelmann: Artist, art therapist and psychotherapist. Former President of the Art Therapy Association Swiss-Romande; lecturer and supervisor of art therapy and psychotherapy trainees in Geneva.
Elizabeth Stone-Matho: Visiting lecturer and clinical supervisor on the art therapy programmes at the Institut de Perfectionnement (INPER) Lausanne and Associazione per lo studio del Disagio Giovanile (ADEG) Turin.
Geoffrey Troll: Sculptor and art therapist, working at the Central Hospital in Dieppe and course co-ordinator (with France-Marie Haeger) of the postgraduate Diploma in Art Therapy at Institut pour Perfectionnement (INPER), Lausanne.
Vera Vasarhelyi: Senior Art Therapist and Lecturer at the Department of Child and Adolescent Psychiatry, United Medical and Dental Schools, Guy's and St Thomas's Hospital, University of London and at Szent-Gyorgi Medical School, Szeged, Hungary.

Also thanks to: Nizetta Anagnostopoulou, Clare Arnold, Maria Belfiore, Juan Corelli, Jhenia and Roumen Gheorghieva, Istvan Hardi, Line Kossolapow, Jacques Lanares, Alexander Marinow, Getie Muntinghe, Rommy Schaap, Marja von Ronkko, Marielene Weber.

Diane Waller,
Goldsmiths College,
University of London

1

Introduction: the need for a European perspective

A question that is bound to arise immediately when looking at the title of this book is: What is Europe and who are the Europeans? The concept of Europe is easy enough in one sense – we look at the map! – but ever since the fall of the Berlin Wall, there has been a shift so powerful that the implications are not yet realized. This becomes very evident in Berlin itself where the 'integration' of East and West is beginning to take place, but it is clear that this process will take a very long time and not be without its traumas as well as excitement. In a market in the old East Berlin, a mixture of people and languages, sounds and smells remind us that Russians, Poles, Turks, Yugoslavs, Italians, Iranians as well as Germans live and work there. In a market in Brixton, South London, we find mainly families of Afro-Caribbean origin, in one in Camden Town, north of the River Thames, there are Greeks, Cypriots, Turks and Irish, and in Whitechapel in East London, along with the long-present Jewish population, there may be Pakistani, Indian, Bangladeshi people. To the west, we find many Irish, Poles and Yugoslavs. All over London, just about every other nationality mingles with the original Cockneys and migrants from other parts of the UK. In Paris, we find Russian emigres from the 1920s, Algerians, Moroccans and Egyptians, as well as people from sub-Saharan Africa.

The issue of 'whose Europe' becomes very clear when we take some of these examples into account. Many European citizens came from non-European backgrounds, originally maybe for work purposes. Often they have been subjected to extreme racism and become very disillusioned by the limited opportunities offered, especially during the recession period, which started during the mid-1980s in western Europe. Some have fled oppressive regimes, civil war and dictatorships and find themselves refugees or asylum seekers. All these changes have considerable implications for health, including and perhaps especially for mental health. At a conference 'Europe without Frontiers: Implications for Health' held in 1992, the Regional Director for Europe of the World Health Organization suggested:

> Another great danger in the present situation [of rapid change] is the effect on the mood of people. For decades the hundreds of millions of people in central and eastern Europe have been anxiously waiting for political freedom, expecting democracy to bring a rapid and tangible improvement in their daily lives. The present desperate economic situation and the prospect in many of the countries – but not all – of a further deterioration before a turn-around can occur, now presents a real danger, undermining support for the new reform processes and increasing the attractions of simplistic solutions. This threatens the social health fabric, increasing the risk of alienation, of the young in particular, leading to criminality, risk of drug abuse, depression and other threats to health.
>
> (Asvall 1993: 10)

If they are unfortunate enough to find themselves needing mental health services, in theory any of these citizens may require or be offered the services of an art therapist. In practice it is unlikely in most European countries at present that they would have access to art therapy. In the future this may change, and it places a great responsibility on our profession, for any form of psychotherapy requires the therapist to respect the client and be open to learning about their lifestyle and cultural context, however dissimilar this may be from the therapist's. I want to state this right at the beginning to make it clear that within Europe the issues of racism and colonialism cannot be ignored. Neither can they be thoroughly addressed in this book, although they are fully acknowledged.

Introduction: the need for a European perspective 3

As to the research for this book, it was initially stimulated by the work I carried out in Bulgaria back in the 1980s, under the auspices of the World Health Organization, when I realized how specific had been the development of art therapy in the UK and in the USA from the 1940s onwards. I was obliged to reframe my thinking about training and professional development in the somewhat ambivalent context of Marxist-Leninist Bulgarian psychiatry (see Waller 1983, 1984, 1996; Waller and Gheorghieva 1990) which raised just about every possible question concerning the theoretical base of art therapy as practised in the UK. In parallel to the Bulgarian project I did some detailed research on the development of the profession in the UK up until 1982 (Waller 1991) and then began a long and exciting quest to see what was happening in this field in the rest of Europe. In 1989 the British Association of Art Therapists (BAAT), which is the UK's professional art therapy association, became involved with the Council for Professions Supplementary to Medicine (CPSM) in considering the implications of the European Directive on the Recognition of Professional Qualifications (89/48/EC) (Commission of the European Communities 1989).

The CPSM was acting as the 'competent body' for carrying out the directive on behalf of art therapists, and it did this in co-operation with BAAT officers. Realizing the complexity of the notion of free movement of professionals across Europe, I attended many meetings organized by the Department of Trade and Industry and saw how well-established professions were trying to grapple with issues of comparability in training and practice. Although there has been little work for art therapists to do so far, given that the Directive only applies where professions are regulated in various countries of the European Union, we need to prepare for the future. The thought of free movement of art therapists was difficult to contemplate given that it appeared there were such differences in the stage of development and even in the definition of art therapy throughout Europe. This problem is not, of course, confined to art therapists. At the same 'Europe without Frontiers' conference mentioned previously, Karin Poulton of the Department of Health said:

> The health care professionals supplementary to medicine constitute a much smaller group [than nurses and midwifery

staff], mainly educated in universities and higher education institutions. These are growing professions and, unlike nurses and doctors, the work of these professions may vary considerably between countries. Some of the work identified as a separate profession by some countries may be subsumed by other professions as part of their work in other countries.

(Asvall 1993: 85)

As we shall see, this last sentence certainly applies to art therapy.

An important and stimulating conference was organized at the University of Leeds in 1993 called 'Facing the European Challenge: The Role of the Professions in a Wider Europe' at which I delivered a paper in a session with the Chair of the Association of Child Psychotherapists (Waller 1994). Our papers and subsequent discussions revealed many common problems to be faced. The child psychotherapists are a very small profession in the UK, regulated within the National Health Service – in fact the only regulated psychotherapy profession – and they have chosen to act as the competent authority for child psychotherapy under the European Directive. They are obliged to deal with the complexities of definition of the term 'psychotherapy' and the considerable differences in training standards throughout Europe. The thoughts I had following this conference proved to be fundamental in shaping this book. Other stimuli were conferences held at Hertfordshire College of Art (now part of the University of Hertfordshire) in the late 1980s and early 90s.

In the course of corresponding with contributors and receiving information from many art therapists and interested others, I have become aware of the rapidly increasing public and professional interest in art therapy in Europe over the past few years – such that I had to decide to stop gathering information or the book would never be finished. I also started to write it before art, music and drama therapy in the UK became state registered (March 1997), so had, rather quickly, to change a great deal of my own contextual thinking to take this major change into account. The book is organized to explore issues that seemed to occur regularly, rather than to be a chapter by chapter description of the state of affairs in various countries.

It is a first attempt on my behalf to explore in some depth the preoccupations of art therapists in Europe, which may well concern others outside Europe, especially in those countries (the majority) where there is yet no profession established. It does not attempt to cover all Europe, which is not to say that in those countries that are not mentioned, or hardly mentioned, there is no art therapy, nor individuals who are working, nor associations formed. Nor does it imply that in those countries that have been examined closely, the situation is necessarily 'good'. Countries of the former eastern Europe are mentioned alongside those of the European Union, although at present the directives only apply to EU countries. The book is certainly not intended to be the definitive view about art therapy in Europe. By way of illustration of how some of the issues identified work out in practice, I have included a good number of examples based on the reported situation in a few countries, chosen for their differing geographical, cultural and political position.

I have also included accounts of the development of art therapy in Switzerland and Ireland as case studies of two small countries which have very different histories, cultures, language and socio-economic contexts. In Switzerland there are three different parts with four languages: French, German, Italian and Romansche, but which are formed into a confederation, and in Ireland there are two separate countries separated by bitter conflict, one part united with Britain and the other a European Union country in its own right. To some extent Switzerland is, or has been, an island within Europe.

For the general theoretical framework of the book, I have been much influenced by Norbert Elias's model of process sociology, and in particular the process model of professions (see Bucher and Strauss 1961) and see the book as part of a process of exploration and partial explanation. One of my aims has been to stimulate debate and to encourage those people who are working in isolation to know that there are colleagues who are interested and may be able to help. Having been intimately involved in the state registration process of art therapy in the UK, I will draw on some UK experience that has led to state regulation. Clearly, having been so involved in this process I tend to think regulation is a good thing for art therapy in that it provides for protection of the public. It imposes limitations on practice and the behaviour of practitioners, which seems to be necessary in the interests of ensuring that vulnerable patients get safe treatment. My personal position is someone who enjoys the collegiate feeling of being part of a lively, dynamic and problematic movement like art therapy, in which many fundamental values are shared with friends and colleagues throughout Europe. The remarkable changes that clients may make through this amalgam of art and psychotherapy, and the rewarding work of sharing in such changes has been inspiring and I believe is at the root of art therapists' wish to promote the discipline. At the same time I am trying to hold on to a sociological position to face the realities, the conflicts and limitations which are bound to be many. It's a challenge!

Part I

Case studies

2

Art therapy in Ireland

Deirdre Horgan

When we speak of Ireland we are referring to two distinct areas, one of which, Northern Ireland, remains within the United Kingdom, whereas the southern part is a republic and a member of the European Union in its own right. These two parts have been divided by a long and very savage conflict, involving religious (Catholic and Protestant) and economic issues. Despite many attempts at bringing about peace, there is still a tense relationship between North and South, between Ireland and the UK. So the conflict goes on, punctuated by truces and cease-fires but with threats of terrorism hanging over the heads of citizens of both parts and on mainland Britain. Whose interests are being served by this conflict and its maintenance? The recent war in the former Yugoslavia led many to comment that Britain still had a civil war on its doorstep and it was not just in the troubled Balkans where neighbours killed each other. Most Irish art therapists have been brought up to face this dangerous situation. They have had to go abroad to train but most have filtered back with the intention of setting up services. It would seem that this is one part of the world where the skills of an art therapist in dealing with anxiety, trauma and bereavement are greatly needed. The following case study by Deidre Horgan shows how the history and context have deeply affected the development of art therapy in both North and South.

Diane Waller

The seeds of plants may be dispersed by wind or animals, or they may be carefully collected and transported by cultivators who nurture them until they flourish. How they develop and spread depends on the type of soil, climate and competition from other species. So it is with new ideas, disciplines and maybe even the emergence of a new profession like art therapy. We can try to encourage growth and development but ultimately there will always be factors outside our control that affect direction and size and shape.

Art therapy has had several beginnings in Ireland, at different times and in different places, but it was not really until the late 1980s that it really took root and began to spread. At present it is finding its own niche in a rapidly changing and developing society and the future remains difficult to predict.

Rita Simon, the first art therapist practising in Ireland, the first person to try and cultivate the beginnings of an art therapy movement, had to start twice. In an interview she describes her reaction on returning to Northern Ireland after 10 years absence.

> It had fizzled out! Charlie Robinson had had a heart attack so he was in no shape to do anything, and others had gone back to their previous work. I had to start again. At that time conditions weren't as favourable as they had been just after the war when rehabilitation programmes and Britain's Health Care system were being redeveloped.
>
> (Coulombe 1995)[1]

The first art therapists in the south of Ireland trained in the United States and returned to work in Dublin. Unlike Simon in Belfast, Sheila McClelland left for England in the late 1980s and Bernadette McClearey (who returned 1984) did not attempt to set up a group or association, but focused on developing their work as individuals initially:[2] 'People have asked me did I feel like a pioneer when I returned from America. No – to me therapy is something quiet that we can only hope will work' (McClearey). Because of the vagaries of partition, art therapists on both parts of the island tended to look abroad for support, training and inspiration rather than to each other. Bernadette McClearey first heard of Rita Simon's work while she was studying in the US with Eleanor Ullman.

While the Northern Ireland Group of Art Therapists (NIGAT) was established in 1976 to provide support and generate awareness of art therapy, it was not until the mid-80s that a small group consisting of two art therapists and two drama therapists was formed in Dublin. Although living in Dublin I am a frequent traveller to Belfast and so the first organization that I became involved in was NIGAT. What I valued most was the opportunity to participate in experiential workshops as well as meeting and networking with others (Horgan 1992).

NIGAT, which developed from the original networking of Rita Simon, has a membership of 75, 13 of whom are qualified. This broad-based structure is a very important aspect of its energy and dynamism. The regular workshop days and newsletter provide fertile ground for people who do want to go on and train to prepare more thoroughly and also keeps the profile of art therapy as high as possible in Northern Ireland. The disadvantage is a common one, that in the context of no formal training or recognition, enthusiastic amateurs may seek to integrate art therapy into their work. But there is no doubt that the open inclusive approach of NIGAT has done much to create an indigenous base for the development of art therapy theory and practice.

The Irish Association of Drama, Art and Music Therapists (IADAMT) was established in 1992 and developed from a core group of arts therapists who had trained abroad and were in the process of establishing their professions in Ireland. Its aims were to be a professional body primarily and so it defined a two-tier membership – professional and associate. Professional membership is only available to those arts therapists who have completed a recognized training in drama, art or music therapy. The challenge is that a small number of qualified therapists are overstretched in providing for their own needs and that of the associate membership. To address this the organization has recently voted to include the associate membership more actively in organizing and running events, attending council and general meetings, but retaining voting rights for professional members.

In the last seven years the number of art therapists has increased dramatically, the small support group in Dublin has evolved into the Irish Association of Drama, Art and Music Therapists and the organizations in the north and south have become more entwined, while retaining distinct identities. Many arts therapists in Ireland are members of both organizations, and did, or do, work on both sides of the border. IADAMT has a regular section in the well-established NIGAT newsletter, which now goes to all members of both associations. A regular exchange involving presentations and workshops is arranged annually. Both associations have appointed someone to liaise specifically with the other. In short, the difference in origin and emphasis has not proved a barrier to the growing relationship between the two organizations. Instead there is a recognition of common goals and interests and workshop days have generated a lot of exciting ideas and fun.

These exchanges are important in establishing the flavour and particularity of Irish arts therapy practice. How stimulating it is to be listening to a colleague relate a case study or present an approach that is happening here and now as opposed to always drawing from a literature which may be written from a very different cultural perspective.

It seems as though the interest and commitment to establishing an identity for arts therapies in Ireland and exploring what that might be in an experiential way is very strong in both organizations. Neither NIGAT or IADAMT have ever felt that it is appropriate to be a regional group of the British Association of Art Therapists (BAAT). Both are committed to a training developing in Ireland and would prioritize its cultural relevance and inclusion of Irish art therapists over its exact location on the island.

Interestingly, this model of mutual support, recognition and common goals/interests has many parallels in the world of the arts, if not in the world of politics. CAFE (Creative Activity for Everyone), the umbrella organization for community arts in Ireland is a 32-county operation, and there is much liaison between the arts councils on both sides of the border. It is almost as though the arts provide a space where people can move more freely and explore identity in a way that is not confrontational or exclusive.

An important decision of the original support group which eventually formed IADAMT was to form one professional association rather than to split into three. NIGAT also includes music, drama and dance movement therapists among its members. What originally started out as a necessity owing to the small numbers of qualified therapists is now seen by the association as a distinct advantage and will undoubtedly be a huge influence on the way art therapy develops both theoretically and professionally in Ireland.

The confidence to work together this way, building on our common interests while firmly holding onto and propagating the belief that each one is a distinct specialization, may have grown from the experience of a number of joint projects undertaken together. I can think of three in which I have been involved:

1 Steps in Expression: Steps in Expression was a day of workshops organized by IADAMT in Trinity College, Dublin. The aim was to promote and publicize the work of arts therapists and it was very successful. A further spin-off was the opportunity it offered arts therapists of different disciplines to work together designing and facilitating workshops which offered an integrated approach to arts therapies.
2 Mutual Supervision Group: The Mutual Supervision Group is a peer supervision group involving art, music and drama therapists that has been operating in Dublin for four years. We have explored different models of supervision and were greatly helped by a workshop organized by IADAMT and facilitated by drama therapist Alida Gersie in 1995. From our experience of being in a group together combined with comparative experience of supervision with psychotherapy and counselling colleagues came an awareness of the richness of media we were using and the potential of the non-verbal processes it offered. From personal experience, supervision with drama and music therapists has helped me to stay with the metaphor the client was using and respond accordingly rather than translate things too quickly into a theoretical framework.
3 Meitheal: Meitheal (a Gaelic word meaning 'cooperative working party') was a further step in exploring the relationship between the arts therapies and the possibilities that this offered for establishing a particularly Irish language of therapy and therapy training.

The idea of advanced or further training in Ireland as part of an ongoing professional development was first mooted as a possible MA model, with supervision and ratification via a recognized training centre in England. The need for such a programme in the context of developing Art Therapy (Postgraduate Diploma) training in Ireland was expressed in my own paper 'Bringing it all back home' (Horgan 1992), in which I said that 'the provision of advanced training for art therapists working here would mean that they could avail themselves of all the job opportunities that such a full-time training would ultimately provide.' At that time (1992) it would have been virtually impossible to establish a career in Ireland and concurrently pay for such a training in England.

Instead, we focused on a self-help solution. Meitheal has its roots in agricultural practice where people banded together to bring in the harvest. We realized that we also needed to pool our resources in order to grow and develop as individual therapists and to explore art work in an independent, co-operative creative framework. A group of 11 – comprising six art therapists, three drama therapists and two music therapists – developed a pilot programme to test the possibilities. Jim Cosgrove and Liam Plant wrote about Meitheal:[3]

> The initial planning meeting identified therapy issues to be explored, and a curriculum was devised. The timetable was agreed on a one day per month basis over six months... Planners and resourcers offered to facilitate and research each curriculum day and costing was organised on a co-op basis... The core feature was that it was an evolutionary process, independent of any institution and growing from an organic skill-share experience.
>
> (Cosgrove and Plant 1994)

Meitheal was very stimulating and exciting; it generated confidence in both individual members and in our abilities as a group. It focused on the richness that was already available within our small population and was the first example of how we had harnessed that for our own development. It explored the boundaries between teacher and pupil, expert and novice, as we all at various stages assumed these roles, exploring unfamiliar media, facilitating or participating in the process. This dynamic is particularly relevant to establishing yourself and working as an art therapist in Ireland, which often demands that you be both expert and beginner at the same time (Horgan 1992).

We learnt how to feed ourselves rather than hunger after the nourishment of our various training courses. Perhaps not surprisingly then, one of the recurrent themes of Meitheal was the potential of the arts therapies to develop a theory from within as opposed to continually seeking validation from other related spheres:

> Words that characterise Meitheal would be:
> Co-operative, non-competitive, non-hierarchical, organic, active, creative, exploratory and validatory. One of the agendas was to establish our sense of separate identity through what we believe is an alternative method of advanced training. Professionally and academically the creative therapies are often validated through the language and framework of verbal psychotherapy... The process of Meitheal enabled us to explore such issues through a creative format of our own devising. This validated for us the distinct qualities inherent in the arts therapies, while examining and acknowledging the value to us of psychotherapy theory and practice.
> (Cosgrove and Plant 1994)

To get a flavour of art therapy in Ireland take a peek at an art therapist activist's diary, or try to arrange a meeting. You would be forgiven for thinking that this is a person with a high stress executive job and little spare time, as numerous evening meetings and even the odd breakfast appointment cram the pages. In reality we survive on a hotchpotch of sessional work and arbitrary rates of pay, and at least half of those diary entries entail work of a voluntary nature seeking to promote the profession. Out of the small number of people working here a smaller number are involved at every level – association, meitheal, supervision, etc. This may seem incestuous, but it is also intimate and bonding, and finally exhausting – 'It's Tuesday... it must be a council meeting'. Since 1994 this small group of dedicated activists has taken the group to association status, writing a constitution, code of ethics, etc.

On 30 November 1995, the fruit of all this labour was celebrated in style by the official launch of the Irish Association of Drama Art and Music Therapists in the beautiful and historical Bank of Ireland Arts Centre, Dublin, the seat of parliament before the Act of Union 1801. The atmosphere certainly felt supportive and affirming as friends and colleagues from the caring professions watched music therapy videos, looked at an exhibition of artwork by art therapists and examined the props from our various areas of work – paints, masks, musical instruments. To coincide with the launch we produced a comprehensive document on arts therapies in Ireland.

The platform was deliberately given to speakers from the world of arts rather than the more established speakers from medical backgrounds, and the speeches were thoughtful and inspiring. Declan McGonigle, curator of the Irish Museum of Modern Art, spoke of the need to bring both art and therapy out of their respective ghettos and see them as part of the centrality of human experience. He placed art therapists in the context of the contemporary movement of artists to work outside the studio. This resonated with many Irish art therapists, including myself, who continue to develop their own artistic identity while working as art therapists.

The launch was certainly the highlight of 1995, but now that our boat is afloat much choppy water remains to be negotiated. It was good to feel the support and enthusiasm of friends but important to realize that it is all too easy to preach to the converted.

There remains no statutory recognition of the arts therapies as professions in health care or education in Ireland. Pay-scales, a professional structure and a recognized training course have all to be established. How these developments take place at a time of cut-backs, emphasis on therapies that can be empirically tested and a general move away from salaried to contractual employment by the public sector is difficult to see.

Work

There are currently about 23 qualified art therapists working in Ireland. The vast majority of these are members of IADAMT or NIGAT or both. There has never been an advertised job for an art therapist so the routes to and types of employment are various.

Most art therapists have to go on a self-advertising campaign, writing letters, producing a leaflet, and doing workshops for prospective employers. Through this they tend to generate sessional hourly-paid work. This type of employment is becoming increasingly common in many areas as the costs to the employer are minimal. Gradually as the art therapist builds up a reputation the need for self-promotion decreases, possibly one job develops into a core job and other sessional or private work can be fitted in around this.

However, the dynamics of the situation are fickle and there is a tendency to take on more work than is manageable because of insecurity in the long term. A small number of hours may be spread over a number of institutions, all with different client groups and dynamics. While this may be a great way to gain broad experience it is tiring and stressful. You have to create your own support systems in terms of supervision, sick pay, holiday pay, etc. and may need insurance cover. It is difficult to include all these costs and remain competitive.

Liam Plant has been working in this way for 10 years and has built up a practice in adult psychiatry. He explained the advantages and disadvantages:

> As a lifestyle it suits young people. As you get older you realize the advantage of more job security. I had two years in the 80s that were a real struggle. I was never tempted to leave art therapy as a profession but I did feel pressurized by economic circumstances.
> (Plant, interview, 1996)

During this time, Liam, like many other sessionally employed art therapists, supplemented his income with work as a teacher or art instructor, often being employed to work in this role with special needs groups. Now the core of his practice is two days with a psychiatric day service who – recognizing the value of his contribution to their programme – gradually increased the hours. Liam stresses the importance of this development as a sessional worker:

> It is important to have an anchor job in terms of support. A job whose function is art therapy in the way one wishes to practise, rather than having a core job as an instructor and then trying to pick the real art therapy jobs on the margins.
> (Plant, interview, 1996)

Having successfully built up and maintained a sessional practice, Liam sees the advantages as broad experience, space to develop private work and do workshops, and a broader range of contacts which continue to bring variety into his work. For example, he is currently involved in offering personal art therapy as an option to students on a postgraduate counselling course in Trinity College, Dublin.

Other art therapists are returning to a post where they hope to use art therapy skills gained while on secondment or career break. Daniel Cullen returned to his job as a probation officer after a three-year career break during which he trained at St Albans. He feels it was an advantage not to be placed directly back in his old post (in the prisons) but instead as part of a team running an intensive probation scheme for young male offenders.

Although there is no mention of art therapy in his job description, the fact that he has been given responsibility to design and develop the creativity module of the scheme is recognition of his new skills. Current programmes for offenders are very influenced by cognitive and behaviour modification approaches, so he finds it quite difficult to introduce a module based on his non-directive art therapy style of working.

Daniel has therefore used the educational potential of team feedback to increase awareness of applications of art therapy and understanding of what he is doing with this module. He feels there is a lot of support and recognition from colleagues, but is realistic about the chances of ever being given an art therapy post in the system. The Probation Service does not have a good record on specialization, although the Probation Board in Northern Ireland has recognized Eileen McCourt (an Irish art therapist, currently working within the probation service in Ireland) as such. Daniel's determination to build things from the grass roots up is evident: 'People who work at the coal-face – if it works they'll use it, regardless of what it's called' (Cullen).

Mary McMahon also found that her training and experience working as an art therapist was very useful when she returned to the coal-face of the classroom a couple of years ago. The art therapist's knowledge of self-esteem and how to foster it is an increasingly valued skill in her role as a primary school teacher. By promoting the medium of art in the classroom she is able to create a different kind of space for children and maximize the potential for empowering and facilitating them within the education system.

She has found that this can have ramifications outside the classroom as well and the perspective of art therapy can be brought to bear on the development of the ethos of a school. She has been encouraged to give talks to parents on developing self-esteem through art and feels there is support from other staff: 'When a few like-minded people get together in a school the emphasis can move from crisis management to a more facilitating approach' (McMahon).[4] In this situation art therapy skills and approaches – although not directly used – can be seen as a catalyst for change in the classroom, school and maybe even the wider community.

There may also be a chance for art therapists to be employed on a more formal basis in educational settings. The Department of Education (Northern Ireland) created posts of teacher–counsellors in 1994 as part of a pilot scheme in inner city schools. If this scheme is successful it may well be extended and teachers trained as art, music or drama therapists would be obvious candidates.

Alternatively, some art therapists have obtained employment as care workers, instructors and teachers in special education, hoping to convert the post or use it to introduce art therapy where there is an obvious need. From personal experience and talking to others, this seems to be a high stress option which generates a lot of internal wrangling within the institution.

Susie Cahn was the first person to create an art therapy post – salaried employment, job description, holiday pay, sick pay, etc. – within an existing organization. Replying to an advertisement for a counsellor with a well-known voluntary organization (the Rape Crisis Centre), she suggested that they take on an art therapist instead. They responded to this imaginatively by creating two half-time posts and offering one of these to Susie: 'I sought out a post as a personal preference and passed over sessional and private work. Financially I wanted a stable income and professionally the advantage of being integrated into a team' (Cahn, interview, 1996).

Susie trained in the United States, graduating with a master's degree. She feels her training gave her a very good grounding, but 'I was still a baby art therapist, confident doing workshops because I was talking to people who knew nothing but doing clinical work. I wanted the benefit of good clinical support' (Cahn, interview, 1996).

She contrasts the dynamics of this with her perception of sessional work:

> As a sessionally employed art therapist I felt I would always be in the selling position rather than being well supported by the team. These are quite conflicting roles. My 'selling' art therapy happened in the interview when I persuaded them not to hire another counsellor but to take on an art therapist and then it was over.
>
> (Cahn, interview, 1996)

She goes on to describe the advantages of being part of a multidisciplinary team:

> At the beginning I was still a bit insecure about skills being borrowed, but by the end of two and a half years there was a common skills sharing from people with psychology, psychotherapy, social work and family therapy backgrounds using a variety of other techniques with the same client base, e.g., hypnotherapy trance work, body work. In the end there was a lovely sharing of skills and a nice eclecticism evolved. My unique skill of art therapy evolved from not being well understood to being highly valued and utilized.
>
> (Cahn, interview, 1996)

The voluntary sector in Ireland has traditionally filled the gaps in services provided by the state (Horgan 1992, Coulombe 1995). Although their budgets are limited they have more autonomy and flexibility in offering employment. At present all art therapists are working through voluntary agencies (Rape Crisis Centre, Our Ladies Hospice, and the lay voluntary hospitals).

However, the real growth in therapy services in Ireland is in the private sector, and a number of art therapists have started practices in this way. Bernadette McClearey returned from the States in 1984, and although there was interest in her skills, there was no funding even for sessional work, and if she had not started working privately she may have had to change career: 'As a painter I was used to "making do" and being resourceful' (McClearey, interview, 1996) These skills helped her in starting art as a self-employed therapist. She also found it of great benefit to have a mentor who had been through similar experiences and cites the influence and support of Fr Michael O'Regan, founder of psychosynthesis in Ireland as particularly important:

> Michael was familiar with the power of art as therapy through psychosynthesis. [He] had known through experience the effort involved in establishing a practice in a branch of therapy previously almost unknown in this country, in his case it had been psychosynthesis, several years previously. He welcomed what I had to offer and became my mentor during those first important steps of establishing my practice here in Ireland.
> (McClearey, interview, 1996)

Through this initial contact Bernadette's skills became known to religious organizations and programmes interested in offering art therapy as a method of personal counselling for those involved in religious life. For a while this formed the backbone of her developing private practice. During these years she also became the first woman counsellor to a seminary in Ireland.

> It is a tribute to their courage and sensitivity to the potential of our work that they opted for a form of therapy that was not mainstream. I was never questioned in my religious affiliations by any employer connected to a religious institution. It was my work that they wanted to know about and my personhood that they trusted. However I believe that my CV and detailed documentation of my qualifications were a critical element in my initial reception into the field of therapy here.
> (McClearey, interview, 1996)

A number of persons from religious orders have since gone on to train and practise as art therapists in Ireland. Undoubtedly this is part of the dialogue between what is new and what exists that influence the theoretical orientation of art therapy in Ireland.

Theoretical influences on art therapy in Ireland

The most discernable influence on art therapy in Ireland is that of Rita Simon. A number of art therapists in Northern Ireland would see themselves as directly practising and passing on a theoretical view of art therapy offered by Simon's work. This emphasizes the art process and considers the style, that is, the way work is carried out as well as the content of the art object.

> Rita Simon's theory of the symbolism of style extends the therapist's information about both conscious and unconscious activity in art therapy. Its centre and starting point lie firmly in the *art*, emphasizing the process of art making as fundamental to therapeutic progress. Attention to style alerts the therapist to possibilities of therapeutic change, however minute.
> (McCourt, interview, 1996)

This influence, however, tends to be geographically specific to Northern Ireland where Rita worked and continues to do workshops. As more people train abroad, the best metaphor is that of the melting pot. Most art therapists who I questioned felt it was too early to define a theoretical orientation for art therapy in Ireland, but spoke enthusiastically about the openness and eclecticism that they experienced.

> It's hard to see any unifying theoretical inputs. Eclecticism rules the day but what does happen here is amazing cross-fertilization of music, art and drama primarily but other disciplines and related areas. It is fertile ground for new thinking and individuality and a high degree of independence.
> (Cahn, interview, 1996)

> Nobody seems to be hidebound by ideology.
> (Plant, interview, 1996)

The fact that most art therapists have to be flexible and independent in order to get work probably fosters an attraction to an eclectic approach as the most practicable: 'The fact that I work with so many different client groups with so many different needs means that the application of a single theoretical approach wouldn't be appropriate' (Plant, interview, 1996).

The theoretical orientation of art therapists working in Ireland will also be influenced by the impact of the existing cultural climate and values on practice. Ireland is still a relatively close-knit society, although presently experiencing enormous social changes. The small population size itself is a factor. Even in the 'metropolis' of Dublin, with all the trappings of a modern European city, the underlying assumption that any stranger may know someone you know is prevalent – and often true. The opportunity and occasion for people in the same therapy group to meet socially is significant as is the incidence of therapist meeting client outside the session. It is a friendliness and intimacy that visitors are attracted to and comment on, finding it quite amusing to be asked if they know John O'Shea who lives in Sydney too!

This expected sense of closeness and relatedness with the other, with its attendant fear of being talked about or disclosing secrets for fear they be publicized, has implications for the therapist–client relationship and within groups affecting the kind of distance or space that can be negotiated and the confidence that can be placed in a confidential space. Journalist and commentator John Waters argues that the type of communication that evolved in a traditional society still affects the public discourse on Ireland as those traditional values and notions of ourselves break down:

> This language was developed so that people could say what they *should* rather than what they *meant* . . . The fact that the destruction of the old culture is being carried out using the same language results in change being a neurotic response to the old rather than the Brave New Ireland we are promised . . . it is being replaced by a depersonalized vacuum, where the word 'progress' limps with a heavy irony and where intimacy is replaced not by tolerance, but by more public forms of invasion.
>
> (Waters 1996b)

In his regular column in the *Irish Times* Waters continually comes back to this theme, warning that the new orthodoxy that is emerging in the name of modernism, progress and Europeanism, is just as stifling and inhibiting of real change as the old:

> The term modern Ireland is an oxymoron. True modernisation is impossible in a climate of pseudo-modernity, for everything is built on lies. Without proper foundations everything turns to dust. The worst instincts rule. We drift along at the mercy of the lowest common denominator. Almost everything is naff, imitative, low-rent. A genuinely modern outlook is impossible, because the past is constantly denigrated and undermined.
>
> (Waters 1996a)

Waters' viewpoint is a response to what has been the mainstream in Irish intellectual discourse for more than a decade – revisionism.

The same period has seen many previously closed doors of Irish life opened for public scrutiny – the family and the Church particularly. This climate of exposure and disclosure of previously taboo areas has fuelled the view of the past as a primitive and dark place with which we are best to break all connections. Writing about recent disclosures of the shocking treatment of orphans in the care of nuns, another commentator, Fintan O'Toole, warns us again of the dangers of any 'nostalgic' view of the past. Watching images of the orphans (now adults) showing how they had to make rosary beads after school, he finds this more disturbing than the revelations of violence also shown on a recent TV documentary because

> These images . . . change forever and for the worse all sorts of memories that seemed stable and comfortable. I remember the feel of the rosary beads in my mother's gloved hand as I held it on the way to Mass. I remember the white shiny rosary beads that I got for my first communion. I remember the dull black ones that my great-grandmother had wrapped around her joined hands on her death-bed. I remember my grandfather's tan coloured beads as he knelt by his bed every night. And now I have to remember that some of those beads, those symbols of order and goodness, were probably placed by fearful little fingers on pieces of wire resting on the open wounds of children . . . These days with so many battles won it is easy to indulge in nostalgia for the old certainties and to forget that what was most certain about them was their naked cruelty.
>
> It is easy to indulge in liberal self-laceration wondering whether we haven't thrown out the baby with the bathwater. It is easy to be too forgiving of the ignorance, corruption and viciousness that were so pervasive as to be virtually invisible. But to give in to any of those temptations is to betray the courage, resilience and life-giving anger of those whose pain was strung on bits of wire to count out such shameful decades.
>
> (O'Toole 1996)

As a therapist what I see in these commentaries is a society struggling and attempting to come to terms with its shadow side. A lot of our notions of ourselves are challenged as our relationship with the past becomes more complex. The tendency is to scapegoat and split rather than attempt to integrate these experiences, however painful.

> Contemporary Ireland floats on a sea of grief. Many, many people are guilty of causing it. This isn't about one nun or group of nuns, though they have much to answer for. But they are scapegoats too, for others still in hiding.
> (O'Faolain 1996)

And perhaps for aspects of ourselves that we all prefer to hide. With so much of the personal becoming political in contemporary Ireland there is a real need for spaces that can allow people to do some of the work of integration and development. I think of the arts as a potential space for expressing, exploring and developing our potential humanity and, of course, the space offered to clients in therapy.

Art therapy – with its particular aspect of non-verbal expression and communication – and the potential to express different meanings with the one image, may be particularly relevant. Certainly the need for such healing spaces is being recognized more and more by the public at large, if not by the funding agencies.

In exploring what factors may affect the future development of art therapy in Ireland, I decided to look outside the profession itself for opinion. I spoke to three doctors working respectively in child psychiatry, adult psychiatry, and hospice. All employ art therapists on a sessional basis and all are aware of the difficulty in obtaining extra funding to extend the use of art therapy in the service they provide.

Paul McQuaid is medical director of the Mater Child and Family Centre in Dublin, providing a multidisciplinary service for children and families with a range of problems, behavioural, developmental and emotional. It is an area where the need for art therapy is certainly recognized but the funding is very limited. The Mater is a large voluntary hospital funded by the state. To introduce something new it is necessary to persuade either the providers of the service, that is, the hospital management, or the purchasers of the service, that is, the State, that it is not just necessary but effective and more necessary and effective than other services.

> The allocation of money in hospitals is so tight that the introduction of new departments (such as art therapy) is often

unthinkable as everyone is working on a shoestring and are overspending their allocations as it is. Most money goes toward wages. Equipment comes second to wages.

(Carmel Murtagh, quoted in Coulombe 1995)

Dr McQuaid sees the need for art therapists to establish their discipline in the public service arena with recognition and grading structure. He also emphasizes the value and potential of research in persuading the purchasers and providers of health care of the value of new therapies, and stresses that pulling energy into a well designed research project now could yield long term benefits for the profession.

Professor Noel Walsh heads a team running an acute psychiatric unit in a general hospital. The unit is run on psychotherapeutic principles and also has a teaching function for medical students and students of psychotherapy. Professor Walsh feels that the link with University College Dublin is vital in maintaining the stance of the unit, which runs counter to prevailing winds in Irish psychiatry. Here he feels the medical model continues to dominate and it is difficult to fund or develop anything that is not empirically provable. He thinks that the development of art therapy in the immediate future will be affected by this climate: There is a tendency to reduce the mentally ill person or patient to biological symptoms, thus neglecting the creative side of the individual and its essential role in the healing process' (Walsh, interview, 1996). However, Professor Walsh feels that there may be a shift in perception in the future as technological advances fail to fulfil their promise in terms of quality of life. With a lot more leisure time, the role of the arts and humanities may have the opportunity to come back into the centre of things. A cultural shift like this would certainly affect the potential role of the arts in health care.

From his perspective in palliative care, Michael Kearney, director of Our Lady's Hospice, Harolds Cross, a turnabout such as this is coming much closer. He works in an area where the fundamental problem is not fixable in the terms of the medical model and therefore a different approach is called for. This approach places the emphasis on healing as opposed to fixing, requires the medical team to stay with the experience, or go into the experience with the patient. He sees art therapy as central to that activity and he feels that the evolution of a more holistic approach in palliative care could be a microcosm of what could happen in all areas of care. Indeed he would see signs of a shift in thinking in the health services, with more emphasis on patient choice and quality of life.

Training

Undoubtedly one of the biggest factors influencing the development of art therapy in Ireland will be the availability of training. Until now there has been no qualifying course available in Ireland, although introductory courses of various types have been run in the North and South (for example, summer schools in Cork and Belfast, a foundation course in Cork, extra-mural courses in Queen's).

The most significant factor in the development of a training in Ireland has been the negotiations between Cork Regional Training Centre and the University of Hertfordshire. Now in its third cycle of foundation course and planning its fifth summer school, Crawford College of Art and Design (CAD) has generated a large group of people well qualified to complete a postgraduate training and, at the time of writing, impatiently waiting for it to start. Their hopes are likely to be fulfilled in the near future as an initially part-time course will be offered in Crawford CAD. Janek Dubowski, Ron Melling and, recently, Alice Byrnes, largely responsible for the initiatives at Crawford, have always argued that training will have a positive influence on the growth of art therapy posts in Ireland and its development and recognition generally – citing the experience of Britain.

The association has remained sceptical of this casual link, pointing to very different conditions in the Britain of the 70s and the Ireland of the 90s, and has warned against too large a course intake initially. The role of IADAMT in the development of training is clearly as consultant and monitor; it is not itself a training body, however there is a vision within the organization of how training could develop and an understanding of it in the context of 'development'.

The course at Crawford will be franchised from the University of Hertfordshire. The obvious advantage of this is that the course is a tried and tested product, which is recognized internationally within the European context. The disadvantage is that the course was developed for particular cultural conditions and *may* need review or regeneration. This option of franchising or buying an existing course document is often contrasted with developing a course from scratch as if the latter were tedious and unnecessary – reinventing the wheel.

Another model that is open to all developing countries is leapfrogging the mistakes and in-built waste that exist in any system and developing from there. This is not reinventing the wheel but finding the best vehicle for your particular terrain. A number of IADAMT members have worked together on ideas around training that would reflect the interconnectedness of art, music and drama therapy in Ireland, and the influences from the various trainings that members have, American as well as British models. Independently, Trinity College Dublin and the Dublin Institute of Education have expressed interest in developing training. It is early days to see whether these ideas have found an institution that can foster them, but they are further evidence of the vitality, resourcefulness and creativity of the arts therapies in Ireland.

Notes

1 Dr Charles Robinson was the medical superintendent in the Department of Psychiatry in Purdysburn Hospital in the 1950s.
2 Rita Simon is a founder member of the British Association of Art Therapists and has been in practice as an art therapist for over 50 years. Sheila McClelland was one of the first art therapists to work in the Republic of Ireland. She trained and qualified in the United States of America in the 1970s, returned to Ireland in the early 1980s and then took up a post as Senior Art Therapist at the Princess Royal Hospital, Haywards Heath, Sussex and as a visiting tutor at Goldsmiths College, London. Bernadette McClearey also trained as an art therapist in the United States and returned to Ireland in 1984.
3 Jim Cosgrove is a music therapist and former chairperson of the Irish Association of Drama, Art and Music Therapists. Liam Plant is an art therapist.
4 This and other quotations in this chapter are derived, unless otherwise specified, from a series of informal interviews conducted by Deirdre Horgan in connection with this book during 1994.

3

Art therapy in Switzerland

Jacques Stitelmann

The Swiss have four official languages and have to take into account the cultural associations of the three main areas that use French, German and Italian – and also an ancient language, Romansche. They have 26 cantons, each with its own character and ways of doing things. Currently, Switzerland is not part of the European Union, and a recent referendum revealed differences in attitude towards the Union in the three main areas. Unless all agree, Switzerland will not join, so it retains a neutral position that is increasingly difficult to maintain given moves towards a common European currency. The fact that Switzerland is not part of the EU means that the various student and staff exchanges open to EU universities and other institutions through Erasmus, Leonardo and other schemes are not available. The development of art therapy in Switzerland reflects this intriguing multicultural mix. Jacques Stitelmann's account is translated from French. As president of the Association of Art Therapists Swiss Romande (ARAET) based in Geneva, he has been particularly active in the French-speaking area of Switzerland.

Diane Waller

The question of language

The French term *art therapie* is a particular translation of the English art therapy. The term *art* in French is different from that in

English. It gives a sense of a set of cultural and aesthetic values, stemming from the history of art, and which have an official place in museums, galleries, collections, schools etc. The term also brings with it an idea of techniques, of knowledge and skills of an artist. In this case we speak of arts with a small 'a' and with an 's'. In the context we are concerned with, we make references to 'fine art' and in the domain of expression this has a capital 'A' and no 's'. Above all the French term has less sense of a creative process than its English counterpart. To explain this we need to paraphrase in French as *processus creatif, expression, expression artistique,* all of which need to be further defined.

In English, the reference to fine arts seems to be limited to the visual arts, especially to painting. In French this term embraces all forms of expression. This is important as a precedent for allowing us to include naturally in French all media (such as painting, photography, video, theatre, dance, music, collage, sculpture, drawing etc.).

The term *therapie* is used in French in two ways: it either means medicine or cure, and finds its roots in the Greek term *therapeia,* which was associated with a philosophy and with a group of men and women who lived in an ascetic community in Alexandria about two thousand years ago. They practised a type of meditative cure using mainly words and human relationships, and believed that human troubles are more psychological than physical, and that speech is excellent in helping to address human beings in their entirety. The noun *therapeia* may be seen as opposite to the Greek noun *iatrike* which is at the root of the term psychiatry, which treats the symptoms and puts human beings and their language in second place in the cure process.

The term therapy is generally associated with another concept which expresses the media used in the cure: psychotherapy, hypnotherapy, balneotherapy, ergotherapy. However, taken on its own, it evokes and refers to a new acceptance of the concept of psychotherapy.

Its use has multiplied in the past few years in words such as *ludotherapie, hippotherapie, naturotherapie.* This gives rise to mistrust and may create the impression that the therapeutic effect originates in the medium and by getting rid of the relational and psychological dimensions and putting to the fore factors external to the person and to relationships; this is a deformation typical of the modern world. The notion of 'psycho' is thus eliminated but also implied, in order to gain some aura of quality or nobility. In any case, it's an expression of real malaise.

In English the term therapy seems to have much larger dimensions than in French, linked to a definition close to 'a relationship which is helpful in developing personal maturity'. This is (not yet) the situation in French. The literal translation of the term may create confusion and bad feeling that many French authors have attempted to avoid or leave behind by creating new concepts, which have, however, not yet found their place in current usage and are only acknowledged within specific schools of thought. Some people (such as Guy Lafargue (1995), originator of the term *art cru,*) think that it is totally impossible to bring together the terms art and therapy to form a single concept, probably because the term art brings with it a notion of radical, social challenge, whereas therapy implies social acceptance.

There is, therefore, a debate fuelled by the issue of the translation of the term art therapy which thrives on the imperfection of this translation. It is a fundamental one that, because it addresses theoretical, technical, economic, and political issues, may allow us to develop our views on our practice and its effectiveness.

Theoretical influences on art therapy in Switzerland

Art therapy in Switzerland is indebted to the early work of Morgenthaler (1921) who stressed the process of artistic expression as a defence mechanism, rather than the expression of a diseased mind, and less directly, to that of Rorschach (1921). Surprisingly, perhaps, the influence of Jung and the Jungian school of psychotherapy is not pronounced and reached Switzerland mainly via English Jungians in the 1980s, rather than through the Jungian training centre in Zurich. Following Jung (1971) Swiss analysts inspired by his thinking would frequently integrate aesthetic creation into the therapeutic approach without, however, usually developing any sort of reflection that might be called art therapy thinking.

Moving to the world of art, the Dada movement was born in Zurich during World War I and then developed in Paris, Berlin and New York. Here we find one of the main contributions to art to come out of Switzerland. In fact, around the Great War, the hopes of socialism and the disillusionment with the immediate post-war period, Switzerland took in refugees from all over Europe. They brought with them the wounds of sociopolitical explosions, and they also brought to the melting pot of Zurich the turmoil of this rejection of European disorder and of bourgeois, military rational logic.

Dada is associated with the pacifist and anarchist movements and some of these participants are associated with psychoanalysis (particularly Otto Gross and Franz Jung). For Gross, psychoanalysis is a revolution which, at the heart of sociopolitical revolution, presents the individual with their own personal history, psychological chains, and neurosis. The Swiss artists of that period were not insensitive to what people were then calling 'the art of lunatics'. At this period of Dada, Reja's (alias Dr Paul Meunier, 1907) book, the first step towards studying this particular form of art, had just been translated into German, and those of Morgenthaler (1921) and Prinzhorn (1922) were in the process of appearing and impatiently awaited by Hans Arp and Sophie Tauber.

Max Ernst, who was planning to write a work along the same lines as that of Prinzhorn, abandoned it in the face of the enormous scope of the publication by the German doctor. Ernst, who would later be a link with Dubuffet (1949) and his *Compagnie de l'Art Brut*, developed techniques such as frottage (where crayon, or other marker, is rubbed over paper placed on an irregular surface), fumage (where marks are made at random on paper by exposing the paper to smoke) or collage in order to provide himself with expressive access to the unconscious (see Ernst 1992). For Daval (1988: 71)

> his creation will always have an autobiographical character. Seeking out the subject and substance of his work from his inner memory, he uses art as a Freudian-type 'analysis'. And it is he who invented most of the automatic techniques of Surrealism, favouring self-discovery through a play of association similar to the analytic method.

Tristan Tzara himself, the originator of the term Dada and main leader of the movement, would never be taken by the passion for madness and its creations, which he considered romantic and outside the scope of art: 'From the point of view of Dada on the other hand, it is a matter of claiming creation as bold, concerted action, undertaken in full consciousness' (Dachy 1994: 173). Tzara even criticized the passion of contemporary artists for the art of 'lunatics'.

Kurt Schwitters, in his Merz paintings and in the continuation of Dada, recovered objects rejected by the world and assembled them into aesthetic compositions. This appeal for materials that had been destroyed, broken and recovered, not only made this post-war process part of such attempts to restore life out of the destruction by using cheap materials, but this salvage of material was also an attempt to express the rejection of illusion in painting. Surrealism, influenced by Freud's theories, was interested in dreams, the unconscious, illogical spontaneous creation. Artistic embodiment was at that time increasingly seen as a process of developing the person of the artist, as a therapy. Let us remember that Andre Breton came from the world of care. There was that desire to lay bare the hidden layers of the person in order to cause fantasy and dreams to flow forth and to cure the man of his imaginings (Muret 1982: 13). Man or society was seen as sick, and art tended to be first the expression and then the purifier, and finally sometimes the therapist.

Following the forerunners and the first wave, a second stage of development in art therapy arose after the Second World War, which broadly issued from three main sources:

- the founding of the International Society for the Study of the Psychopathology of Expression (SIPE);
- the influences of the practitioners originating from the USA and, to a lesser extent, from England;
- the sociocultural and artistic movements of the 1960s.

The SIPE (in French the Societe Internationale de psychopathologie de l'expression, deriving from the French society of the same name) responded to a need after the world conflict to recreate conditions for international exchanges based on common pursuit and cultural interests. Conferences were regularly organized and articles and books published. Switzerland's involvement was essentially through the activities of Alfred Bader, whom I will discuss later.

The English influence was very marked after the Second World War and the American model became a prime example in psychiatry, among other disciplines. From the 1970s, the humanist movements arrived in Switzerland. English psychoanalysis and the Kleinian schools also influenced practitioners in French-speaking Switzerland.[1]

Finally, the revolutionary sociocultural and artistic movements of the 1960s hit art therapy practices and theories in Europe and in Switzerland too, in full force, while also pushing forward the art end of art therapy in its revolutionary function and its dimension of creative process.

These three influences would cross the different practices and current teachings, but not without posing a number of problems from a sense of belonging to a complex field of practice.

Alfred Bader

To return to one of the paramount figures in art therapy in Switzerland, Alfred Bader, it is thanks particularly to his bilingualism that he has achieved this prominence. This has enabled him to study the writings of the two main national languages of Switzerland, French and German. His historical texts and his lectures at the SIPE during the 1960s and 70s, as well as the creation of his Cery Hospital workshops are remarkable. The workshops were, for him, mainly intended to support the ability of some patients to produce art rather than dwell on morbid symptoms, and secondly to encourage a psychotherapeutic approach.

According to Bader, before the 1940s, some hospitals used to allow or sometimes facilitated the free expression of patients partly because it kept them occupied. A second stage occurred in which, with the use of psychotropic drugs and improvements in psychotherapies, one saw a reduction in the seriousness of the symptoms and also a process of free expression. Then, with the idea of socializing patients or reintegrating them into society, and the improvement in curative techniques, the workshops became not only places of occupation or of art-oriented teaching but genuinely able to provide care and well being. Bader thought that the benefits came through free expression and creation and not through analysis of the content or the relationship with the therapist.

As early as the 1970s Bader was compiling a long list of workshops in psychiatric hospitals, the majority centred around occupation and run by people trained in occupational therapy, along didactic lines. The general aim was to make the patients aware of their creative abilities and to increase their self-awareness. The idea of mobilizing the creative potential of patients was there right from the initial workshops, which were usually run by artists. Very quickly, from the 1960s onwards, training centres came into being (between 1975–80 in Switzerland) to train the facilitators of such workshops in artistic and psychotherapeutic terms. Sometimes the workshops seemed to be fine arts workshops, others resembled group psychotherapy sessions whose artistic creations were interpreted in terms of dreams or fantasies. Sometimes they involved patients copying paintings.

Bader noted there was no consistency in these practices. The workshop he created at Cery, near Lausanne, has existed since 1963. His definition of it was radically different from that of ergotherapy (occupational therapy). There was no doctor, pastor or artist and the contact with the patient came from outside and had no psychiatric nor artistic training. This person was responsible for the materials, facilitated access to various media, prepared the tea and acted freely as needed. He or she built up a friendly relationship with the patients without forcing anyone to paint or doing any counselling. The aim was to create a recreational atmosphere. Bader felt it was important that patients didn't feel they must produce something but that they felt unconditionally accepted as they were. If the facilitator had no expectations, it freed the patients from the pressure of creating beautiful things and meant that the facilitator was interested in the people rather than what they had created. Regular attendance was the desired objective and Bader made the groups up by combining various pathologies. He used quick, light yet rich and diversified technical approaches. There were no prior instructions, either artistic or therapeutic.

The therapeutic dimension lay in the possibility of enabling free creativity and relied very little on cathartic effect. As a general rule group work was suggested, since it relieved the patient's sense of isolation, reduced fear and facilitated communication. Bader attached significance to the post-creation discussion. Analyses of the content and the transferential process could be made by the patient's therapist and taken up in one-to-one psychotherapy.

Bader considered one-to-one art therapy as a non-specific therapy for psychoses. The technical learning that happened as the sessions went along seemed to him useful in enabling the patient to make full use of his or her creative potential. Artistic expression within this framework was to be understood as communication to the therapist, who would not interpret the content but rather focus on the transferential element. Bader noticed that, whereas some time before, the expression of schizophrenics had been perceived as sick, at that time it could be considered as an attempt to defend against the frustrations and indifference of the real world, as a healthy attempt on the patient's behalf to protect himself and to cope.

Jolande Jacobi is an important Swiss therapist who at the start of the 1970s developed thought on obsessional disorders and the way they figured in the paintings and drawings of several of her patients. They were remarkable for the presence of stereotypes, representation of genital, urinary and anal parts, and by latticework (*grillage*). She combined the work of free analysis of paintings with a Jungian analytical approach.

Michel Thevoz actually set himself clearly and energetically against art therapy but holds a place of paramount importance, if only because of his extensive research and the alternative viewpoint he presents. A representative of the 'art brut' movement and curator of the museum of the same name from the time it opened in 1975, Thevoz not only holds the values and ideas on art brut expressed by Dubuffet in the immediate post-war period, but has developed them through a number of works since 1975. To give a quick resumé, art brut involves the creations of people who are little or in no way influenced by the culture of their society. It is can either be simple or sophisticated but the artists do not have any training. Waste, or non-traditional art materials are often chosen, and Thevoz is particularly fond of studying the dimension of natural writing and the creative diversions made by these virtually 'unculturized' people.

In a polemical article on art therapy, Thevoz criticizes the position of workshop facilitators as volunteers and a mercenary attitude towards objects created in art therapy workshops. He has doubts from the outset about the reality of an artistic, or even therapeutic, dimension to these activities:

> We are acting in other words as a coloniser, we collect these
> works as if they were valued spices, for sure, but according

to culinary or artistic norms that remain ours. The handicapped are the unwilling stars or the hostages of an artistic situation which is lost on them.

(1993–4: 434)

Art therapy for Thevoz heralds the death of art:

Art, like sexuality, loses its attraction when it is prescribed like health exercises. That is the dilemma: or else therapy really works, but by neutralising the negativity, asociality or individual dissidence which are the very impulse of artistic expression.

(1975: 434)

These are arguments with which art therapy must continue to engage.

In terms of art therapy publications, Marc Muret's *Les Art Therapies* (1983) attempts to give a history and to erect theoretical and practical milestones for the various art therapies. We should note also the regular publications since 1987 by Fachverband fur gestaltende Psychotherapie und Kunsttherapie (GPK), a German-Swiss association based on the coming together of artistic mediation psychotherapists, through its journal *FORUM*.[2]

Professor Luban-Plozza, in the Ticino (Italian speaking) canton, organizer of the Balint meetings and father of the Ascona model, also supports the field of art therapy through publications as well as by founding an international art therapy association with other German-speaking practitioners. French-speaking Swiss practitioners such as Ursula Tappolet, a Jungian analyst, or Anne-Lise Louca are involved through articles in the French journal *Art et Therapie*, run by Jean-Pierre Klein.

Finally, in 1992, in the English-language journal *Inscape*, Nina Robinson attempted a brief description and analysis of the Swiss situation with regard to art therapy by interviewing German-Swiss practitioners and teachers. She states that in 1978, Esther Dreyfuss Katan, trained in the USA, became the first art therapist taken on in Switzerland by a hospital, where she was working with cancer patients, although art therapy existed well before then at numerous private and institutional locations.

Robinson differentiates two currents that took shape in Switzerland between 1970 and 1995: the first being a German-speaking one of German-speaking Swiss psychotherapists and psychiatrists interested in art, who integrate it into their work without developing specific theories and practices but, inspired by the SIPE, approach the image, its conception and content like fantasies and dreams through psychoanalytic interpretation. The International Association in Basel has its roots in this field. The second, 'Maltherapy', was inspired by Arno Stern from Paris, who taught very early on in Switzerland. The principles of Stern, who distances himself from therapy, are clear: no interpretations, specific tools, repetitive and enclosed (*clos-lieu*) setting. Robinson concludes by observing and deploring the fact that, in Switzerland, art therapy is developing under the wing of other professions. Most people trained continue to teach a basic skill while adding a specialized tool, art therapy. Under these conditions, she comments, private practice is increasingly difficult.

Financing art therapy in Switzerland

There may be three financing systems:

1 The patient pays for his or her own art therapy.
2 Sickness insurance covers part of the treatment.
3 The Office Federal des Assurances Sociales (OFAS) Federal Social Security Office, finances recognized institutions and the educational and rehabilitative psychological treatment activities they propose for disabled beneficiaries unable to work for a living.

Since Switzerland does not have a well-developed social security system, art therapy will depend on the organization within which it is practised and the training of the practitioner.

Art therapy may be carried out within two different frameworks, privately and in a state institution. Privately the system is simple. In most cases, patients must pay for the sessions themselves without social security or sickness insurance support. In 1994 a training institution was able to get its training programme recognized by an association of psychotherapists (Association Suisse des Psychotherapeutes, ASP). Hence it will be able to allow some of its members with university training in social science and psychology, and who have additional intensive training, to become recognized and partially reimbursed through sickness insurance companies. This is already the case for the very few practitioners who lecture as psychotherapists and include art therapy methods in psychotherapy. In an institution, art therapy may be subsidized by the OFAS within the framework of educational or therapeutic programmes; on the other hand, practitioners are, with very rare exceptions, engaged straight away in posts such as social workers, youth workers, nurses, ergotherapists, psychologists and even artists.

The sickness insurance system in Switzerland is currently undergoing radical change and in the short or medium term it would be wise to aim for our practices in art therapy to be recognized. Four courses seem possible for this:

- By means of psychotherapy as a specialty and through the recognition of the ASP or Federation Suisse des Psychologues (FSP) or Federation des Medicines Helvetiques (FMH), then by the sickness insurance companies, following the route taken by one of the German-Swiss training institutes.
- By means of the model created by the anthroposophists who, within the framework of insurances supplementing the basic sickness insurance, were able to get partial reimbursement for curative painting costs.
- By means of reimbursement from sickness funds for ergotherapy-type care (with the risk of diversion and professional annexation if that were the only route followed).
- By creating and at last structuring the regional associative workshops and getting them recognized by the OFAS after they have been running for a year or two.

The most realistic course might be to follow these four routes simultaneously, each being able to be adapted to different situations with regard to practitioners and to clients and patients.

Training courses currently in existence in Switzerland

I contacted 15 training institutions in Switzerland that have been active over the last few years. I asked them to let me have information on their courses. Seven replied and are still in operation. It seems that a number of others may no longer be operating.

Here are a few pointers from the analysis I made on the basis of their documentation and of the replies I got from a short questionnaire.

Theoretical orientation

- Five centres refer to the humanistic vision as a whole.
- Five refer to psychoanalysis or at least one or two of its thinkers.
- Four refer to Jung.

It is interesting that none of these sources mentions any theoretical artistic example as a fundamental source or base. Is it that they are essentially intended for professionals in the helping field and psychology? Or else is it that the artistic example is approached more as a 'neutral' theoretical tool? Or even that this aspect of the question has not yet been sufficiently thought through? There is an almost general reliance on conventional artistic techniques: painting and drawing on the one hand, theatre, dance and psychodrama on the other.

Functional links and organizational supports

- Two of these centres (those training the largest number of students) became associated during the early 1990s with universities – one in the United States, the other in England – the qualifications granted being recognized by these universities.
- One programme is part of an international system of French origin.
- Two of the training centres offer a programme specific to art therapy among several specialization programmes within the helping field.
- One centre is part of a psychiatric institution.
- Four are directly linked with a private centre which also offers workshops to the public.

Teachers' countries of origin

More than half the teachers are not Swiss but practise and teach mainly in the USA, England and Germany, France or Belgium and come for one or two seminars. Two of the programmes are run by people resident and practising abroad. The courses based on the universities in the USA and England call most upon foreign tutors.

Duration of training programmes

There is a great variety in the length of the programmes since they range from one year to four and a half years depending on the level offered and the intensity of demand from the student.

Explicit aims and objectives of the programmes

Five broad outlines emerge from the seven programmes:

- Personal and formative experience in a broad sense is mentioned twice.
- Continuing education not leading to a formal qualification is mentioned twice.
- Specialization supplementing basic training in the helping field in its broad sense is mentioned six times.
- Psychotherapy through artistic mediation is mentioned twice.
- Art therapy or art psychotherapy as a profession in itself is mentioned three times.

The areas of training offered

I had asked the training institutions to let me know by specific area what sort of training they offer, limiting this to four areas: using oneself as a case study for the method; practice in facilitating workshops; supervision of practice in facilitating workshops; theoretical and methodological teaching.

- The percentage of course time involving using oneself as a case study in relation to the total number of hours varies between 100 and 5;
- The percentage involving practice in facilitating varies between 0 and 60;
- The percentage involving supervision varies between 0 and 15;
- The percentage involving theoretical teaching varies between 0 and 60.

Only the component involving using oneself as a case study is mentioned in all the programmes as an obligatory part of the training.

These results reveal incredible diversity and even a certain amount of inconsistency which shows, apart from the newness of this professional field, that these institutions are certainly not training people in the same practices. The programmes appear to be structured according to the ideas of the people running the training institutions and according to the personal inclinations and capabilities of the people doing the training. It would seem highly useful and necessary that the professional associations should define the minimum curriculum standards.

The current practical situation

In French-speaking Switzerland, where the enthusiasm for art therapy is more recent than in German areas, most practitioners are still currently undergoing specialized training. The majority are professionals from the helping fields such as teaching, education, social work, nursing, ergotherapy and psychology but a small number come from an art-based training. A tiny number (having studied in the USA) are trained solely in art therapy, without having gone through any prior training in the arts or helping fields.

The largest number of practitioners do not practise art therapy full time, but are in general committed to it on the basis of a basic training course and facilitate a few hours part-time at art therapy workshops. Problems are caused, and will continue to be caused, by the shortage of places for professional training, of placements for students undergoing training, and of available posts once training is completed.

The fields for practising the interface between art and therapy seem to me to divide into three:

- psychotherapy through artistic mediation; this is a specialization within psychotherapy;
- the therapeutic expression workshop or art therapy workshop; this is a specialization of the helping professions outside psychotherapy;
- art therapy: this is a practice still in the process of definition; it may be compared to either of the models above, but the main

feature of it is that it refers to a profession in itself, whereas the others refer to a specialization and to a specific practice within the framework of a basis profession.

ARAET

Since December 1993, French-speaking Switzerland has had an association, the Association Romande Arts et Therapies (ARAET), a regional association (of which the author is chairman). We have restricted this association to the French-speaking region for reasons of organic development and practical linguistics. ARAET has set itself the aim of representing all orientations of the art therapy interface, promoting further education, encouraging research, disseminating our ideas to the public, fostering practice–theory exchange, collaborating with all partners in order to promote the status, working conditions and wages of art therapists and expression workshop facilitators, establishing and defending the titles of art therapist and expression workshop facilitator, and collaborating with professionals in closely related disciplines. ARAET currently has nearly 100 members and is in the process of defining minimum levels for, and essential areas and stages of, training.

Prospects for the future

The future for the art–therapy interface in Switzerland seems to me to be marked by three main problems:

1 Multilingualism in Switzerland and the cantonal structuring of the institutions facilitates divisions and ignorance of what others are doing. It also hinders communication.
2 The need to depend upon professions with different bases to get its practices recognized before, possibly one day, a new profession is recognized. This reliance on different professions risks giving rise to conflicts of power and orientation that might have less to do with the specificity of our practices than with the conflicts between these professions themselves.
3 The newness of the structuring of our practices and the weakness of the Swiss sickness insurance support system means that the benefits for these practices are more or less non-existent.

This future may be constructed upon a basis of two major foundations:

1 receptivity to Germanic, French and English cultures;
2 reliance upon a basic profession, generally in the helping field as background training offers some quality assurance.

The following are some of the main issues still to be resolved:

1 The recognition of a new profession, art therapy, does not seem feasible in the short and medium term, although this must be one of the aims of the professional associations.
2 Within the framework of basic professions, it is fundamental to have art therapy recognized as worthy of respect, time and money.
3 The complexity of the art–therapy interface calls for the formation of flexible, intricate associative systems able to enrich themselves from conflicts without being torn apart by them.
4 As far as training courses are concerned, the professionals should, through their associations, define minimum frameworks.
5 Contemporary expressive techniques, curiously little used in our practice, should be explored.
6 Specific research into our practice should be carried out.

Notes

1 The Kleinian school is a branch of psychoanalysis stemming from the work of Melanie Klein. This is also known as the 'Object Relations' school and is, along with the work of D.W. Winnicott, influential on British art therapists. (See Klein 1959.)
2 *FORUM* (1985–1994) was a journal of the Association for Gestalt Psychotherapy and Art Therapy and was produced in Bern.

Part II

The profession

4

Definitions, limits and boundaries

For the purposes of this book I use the term art therapy to apply to visual art therapy (although this in itself poses problems). This position reflects the situation in Britain where there are four arts therapies: art, dance, drama and music, all with their own training and professional organizations. There are nevertheless many links between the professions, notably with art, drama and music, which have all worked together since 1990 to become state registered. In 1989 the Department of Health appointed a music therapy and art therapy advisor, but for an unknown reason no drama therapy advisor. There is a chair's committee of all four professions, a research group, groups exploring the particular needs of employers (for example prison service, education), a race and culture group, and instances of a representative of one arts therapy acting as an external examiner for another arts therapy course or supervising postgraduate students. There is an All Wales Network of Arts Therapists, an Irish Association of Arts Therapists and instances of local arts therapists getting together and organizing joint activities. Still, the arts therapy professions strongly retain their autonomy, especially in terms of education and training, and have come together as a single profession only for the purposes of state registration where they have formed a Federal Arts Therapy Board. I want to emphasize this point because in the Netherlands, for example, these professions are known as creative therapy and are much more closely linked in terms of training and professional development, beginning with initial, undergraduate training and continuing thereon. Close comparison reveals fundamental differences in approach so that the equation of Dutch creative therapy with British arts therapy is misleading (see also Chapter 9).

In Britain, it seems as though the term art therapy was first used by the artist Adrian Hill in the early 1940s to describe his painting classes in a sanatorium in the south of England. It was also used in the USA around that time. Most British art therapists working today would accept that art therapy is a form of psychotherapeutic intervention in which the patient is encouraged to make painted or other visual images, using basic art materials. Such images can be used to communicate emotions and states of mind that may be difficult or even impossible to express verbally. Some art therapists maintain that it is the involvement in the process of visual creativity that aids integration of the personality, and is therefore healing. Others consider that the relationship of the therapist, patient and the artwork, and the ensuing resolution of transference material are essential contributors to the successful progress of therapy. Several authors have explored the particular role of the transference in art therapy, notably Schaverien (1991).

The way in which art therapy has been understood among professional colleagues and the general public has often not been as described above. Indeed, up till this year (1997) the UK Department of Health still had no 'official' definition, but referred to art therapists as being 'responsible for organising appropriate programmes of art activities of a therapeutic application with patients, individually or in groups' (DHSS 1977). There is clearly a difference between 'organizing art activities' and practising in a way that may be closely allied to dynamic psychotherapy. In 1997, anticipating state registration, the National Health Service Executive, working with the arts therapies professional associations, produced a careers leaflet that is an up-to-date description of the practitioners:

> Arts therapists are specialists in a process which combines either visual art or drama or music with therapeutic models. Their fundamental aims include alleviating emotional distress and improving quality of life. The arts therapies are akin to counselling or psychotherapy, and require the therapist not

only to be an experienced practitioner in his or her chosen art form but also to be trained to assist people who are suffering a range of distressing or disabling conditions. Arts therapists work with children and adults, from the very young to the very old, with clients who may be going through temporary life difficulties to those who are chronically mentally ill or suffering from terminal illnesses. They also work with children and families, and practise both with individuals and with groups.

Specifically about art therapy itself, the leaflet says:

> The process of art therapy involves a transaction between the creator (the patient) the image or artefact and the therapist. As in all psychotherapy, bringing unconscious feelings to a conscious level and thereafter exploring them, holds true for Art Therapy, but here the richness of artistic symbol and metaphor illuminate the process.
> (Department of Health 1997)

We can see that since 1982, when art therapy was first regulated by the UK Department of Health, there has been a major change in definition, from 'activities' to a 'psychotherapeutic process'. There still remains much to be done to inform other professionals and the general public, however and art therapists are devising appropriate referral systems so that colleagues and patients understand the nature of the treatment on offer and do not anticipate being taught to paint, for example, or 'having their minds taken off their problems' which may be (erroneous) reasons for referral.

In order to describe more clearly the nature and function of art therapy as a treatment, a suggestion was made to the British Association of Art Therapists' annual general meeting in 1991 to rename the profession 'art psychotherapy' thus incorporating all elements of the process: the patient, the image and the therapist and their interrelatedness and to avoid confusing the process with 'art activities'. This proposal led to fierce, sometimes angry debates among the members of BAAT, resulting in a referendum (1992) which showed that at that time a majority still wanted to retain the title art therapy for the profession. However, a sizable minority preferred art psychotherapy and indeed the qualifying programme at Goldsmiths College is entitled Diploma in Art Psychotherapy and many members now refer to themselves as art psychotherapists.

One of the issues which concerned BAAT members is that by making such a clear link with psychotherapy the art-making process might be devalued. The belief in the healing value of art is a central one for most British art therapists, the majority of whom come from a background in art and design where their primary identity was formed. Psychotherapy is perceived by many members as a verbal, white, middle-class, alien (and often elitist) process, and art psychotherapy seen as one in which images are brought in as an adjunct to the main aim: verbalization of unconscious feelings and resolution of transference issues. The term art psychotherapy thus evokes for some people a sense of art-making as secondary, whereas in practice it should mean integrating art-making more fully into a therapeutic relationship. This debate has been healthy in highlighting differences of approach within the profession itself which in its earlier, formative stages, would have been hard to acknowledge. The state registered designation will be Arts Therapist followed by the appropriate modality, that is art, music or drama, so it is quite possible that those people who feel strongly can identify themselves as a State Registered Arts Therapist (Art Psychotherapist). Later on, when discussing the position elsewhere in Europe (Germany for instance) we shall see that there are similar differences of approach, but these have yet to be incorporated into a single association which represents all views.

For many members, being identified as a profession supplementary to medicine has not been very agreeable, but this feeling has largely disappeared due to the current revision of the Professions Supplementary to Medicine Act 1960 – when the professions registered at that time were considered to be 'supplementary' or 'auxiliary'. The new Act will dispense with this term and the new council is likely to be called the Health Professionals Council, or something very similar. An important proposed element in the new Act is the protection of title. This means that nobody would be able to call themselves an art therapist if they were not on the state register. Should they do so, they could be prosecuted. Currently, only the term 'state registered' is protected. It is still not uncommon, despite 15 years of NHS regulation, for people

Definitions, limits and boundaries 51

who have no training in and very slight knowledge of art therapy – or art for that matter – to refer to themselves as art therapists, such a move is very welcome.

Such a protection of title seems very far away, as far as the situation in Europe is concerned. At an ECARTE conference in Ferrara, Italy in 1994, Truss Wertheim, then vice president of the Dutch Association of Creative Therapists, drew attention to the problem:

> Often the lack of structure and inconsistency is demonstrated in art therapy literature and at conferences and symposia. Contemplating the diversity of subjects displayed in titles of papers and workshops, one is left with the impression that the field of art therapy has no boundaries. Chosen theoretical and/or political directions, having great impact on further development of the profession, are seldom made explicit, yet they do have big consequences for the profession's outline. Nevertheless there are fundamental differences between particular tracks of approach.
> (1995: 32)

She goes on to discuss the identity of the art therapist in Europe, asking: who are the practitioners and what do they call themselves? Importantly, she draws attention to the hierarchical status or theoretical base of art therapy:

> In Holland one finds 'creative therapists in visual art' (*beeldend kreatief therapeuten*) and 'art therapists' who reject the term creative, because they reject a multimodal approach. Also there are 'artistic therapists' (*kunstzinnige therapeuten*) a name which refers to an anthroposophic approach and finally there are creative psychotherapists, a name used by psychotherapists and psychiatrists using art.
>
> In the UK where art therapy is state validated, a distinction is made between 'art therapists', 'art psychotherapists' and 'analytical art psychotherapists'. In Germany there seems to be a differentiation between art therapists (*Kunspsychotherapeuten*) art psychotherapists, (*psychotherapeuten arbeitend mit künstlerischen methoden*) psychotherapists using art, (*gestaltungtherapeuten*) creative therapists and (*kunsttherapeuten*) art therapists.
> (1995: 33)

Wertheim's view is confirmed by all the contributors to this book and indeed by the small amount of literature available on the state of the discipline in Europe.

Defining art

There are not only problems over the definition of art therapy, or art psychotherapy, but also over 'art' within Europe, and this affects the description of art therapy. Vera Vasarhelyi discovered this when introducing a new programme in Hungary:

> As my colleagues and I were in the process of translating from English to Hungarian, it became obvious that the term 'art' was even more ambiguous than it is in English. It carried not only the burden of aesthetic values attached to it – a misunderstanding we often encounter as art psychotherapists ourselves, where we are perceived as providers of a creative outlet for patients marking time in institutions – but also as a much too general and imprecise a word.
>
> Art in Hungarian means any form of art, music, drama or dance. It therefore opens up another source of confusion concerning identity by suggesting that it is a kind of 'creative therapy'.
>
> After careful consideration, I felt that the term 'Visual Psychotherapy' would express most clearly the essence of a therapy where the visual image is a direct reflection of internal, unconscious processes, untainted by external attributes such as skill or conformity to a socially acceptable aesthetic criteria.
>
> (Vasarhelyi 1992: 21)

In Finland, there has been training in visual arts therapy since 1974 at the university of Industrial Arts in Helsinki, supervised by the university itself, the Finnish Association of Art Therapists, and other institutes. We note that the title includes both visual and arts. Wita Szulc (1995: 11) writing about an art therapy training in Poland, tells us that:

> The Polish authors use the term *art therapy* referring to creative art therapy in general, that is to 'the use of art and other visual media for therapy or treatment', as well as to music

therapy, dance therapy, drama therapy, and – perhaps to your surprise – bibliotherapy (Janicki 1990).

I myself use a general term, culture therapy. This is because all those therapies use cultural means as therapeutic tools. I refer here to the theory of culture meaning symbolic culture and not anthropology of culture, the art being the most representative branch of symbolic culture . . . Culture therapy, according to my definition, is one of many actions directed to humans and their environment, directed to improve the quality of life and aimed at recovering and powering health.

This concept of 'cultural therapy' is taught by Dr Szulc in postgraduate medical schools and, in common with Bulgaria, Yugoslavia and Hungary, art therapy is seen as a treatment to be carried out by the medical profession or occasionally by teachers. It is seen as a diagnostic and therapeutic technique, applied in hospitals, schools and institutions for children with special needs.

Definitions complicated by language

An even more complex question of definition arises from the different languages themselves and it seems in particular, the French language and the meanings of art and therapy as concepts (see Chapter 3). I think that a similar problem applies to Italian, on the basis of interviewing approximately 100 entrants to various introductory art therapy programmes who when asked about their art interests and experience, cited every form of visual, musical, dramatic art, dance, films, making furniture, studying icons, going to concerts, restoring paintings, visiting galleries. Very few had actually engaged in any visual art practice.

The problem of other professionals claiming to 'do art therapy' without any training or experience is unfortunately rather common. It was also the situation, Karin Dannecker recalls, as described by Elinor Ulman in the USA, in 1975:

Many refer to certain professional and volunteer workers as art therapists, even though no similar educational preparation, no set of qualifications . . . binds these people together. Possibly the only thing common to *all* their activities is that the materials of the visual arts are used in some attempt to assist integration or reintegration of personality.

Problems concerning the meaning of the term art therapy is found in Austria, where as in Germany, the term *Kunsttherapie* is used. Wolfgang Mastnak (personal communication) explains:

> There is no official or legal definition of art therapy in Austria. Still the term 'Kunsttherapie' (Kunst = Art) is handled with a distinct meaning which derives from therapeutic tradition as well as from the use of the word 'art therapy' abroad. Art therapy in Austria stands for the entirety of therapeutic interventions based on creating and experiencing images. The meaning of 'therapy' includes psychotherapy (e.g. with neurotic clients), psychiatric and neuropsychiatric intervention (e.g. with psychotic in- and outpatients) particular pedagogic practice with handicapped children, geriatric applications, psychosomatic prophylaxis (e.g. concerning stress-related diseases) and the wide range of rehabilitation.
>
> The essential idea of art therapy focuses on the artistic process. This means that art therapy need not take its roots from any other (e.g. psychological theory). There is no pre-existing theory compulsory upon the development of new art therapeutic concepts.

In reflecting on the above examples of definitions, it is perhaps useful to remind ourselves that in the UK and in the USA, the roots of art therapy are strongly placed in the art education movement of the 1930s, which actually stemmed from Franz Cizek's child-centred work in Austria and was taken forward by such pioneers as Marion Richardson in the UK and Florence Cane in the USA. Although art education varied greatly in the level at which it was taught in the UK, painting as self-expression was usually found in nursery and primary schools, and art was taught as a practical subject involving materials and methods. In many parts of Europe, including Eastern Europe, art in the curriculum meant art history, or study of classical forms. Practical art work was carried out, if at all, in after-school classes. It can happen that participants in workshops in, for example, Bulgaria, Hungary and Italy, have had no experience whatsoever in handling art materials and their knowledge of art remains on a theoretical level.

It would seem to be the norm, then, across Europe, for there to be a problem with the term art therapy, given that usually art encompasses visual art, drama, music, dance, literature. Also, art

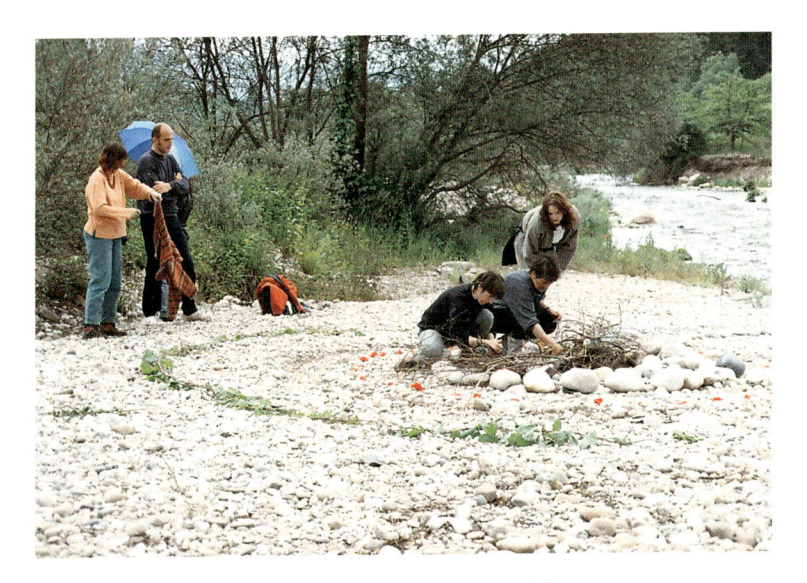

Foyer group work with wood, stone, leaves and fire
© J. Stitelmann

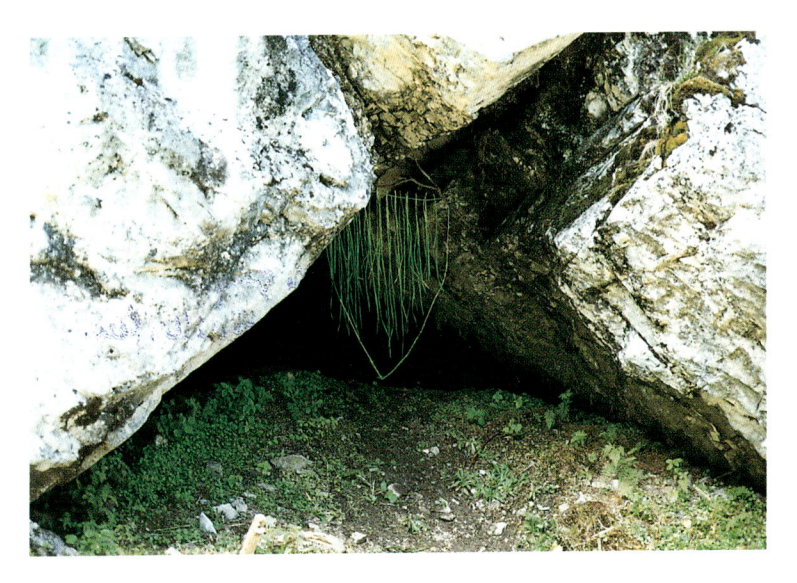

'Woman' – stones, cave and leaves
© J. Stitelmann

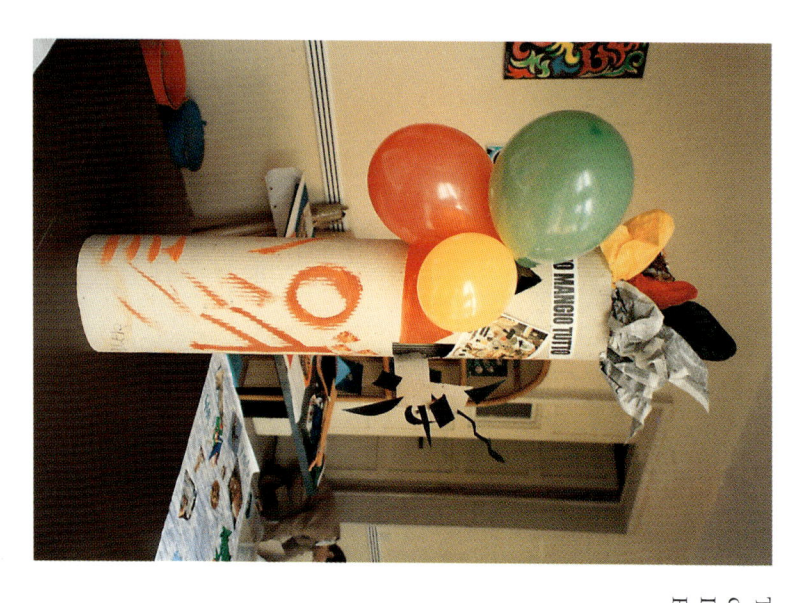

Three dimensional collage, Centro Italiano, Rome
Photo: Dan Lumley

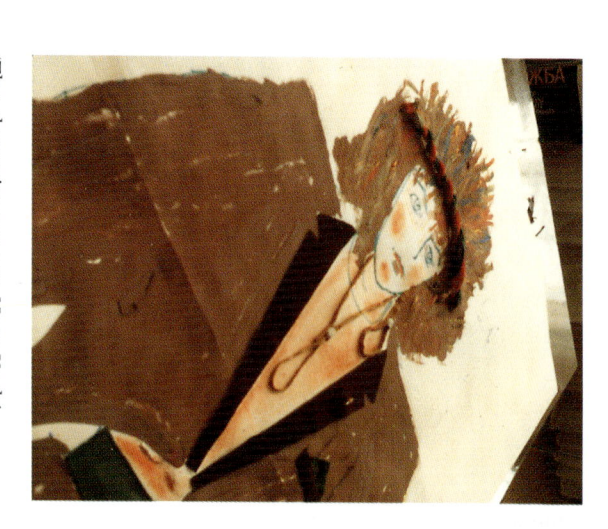

'The therapist goes to New York', Varna, Bulgaria, student
Photo: Dan Lumley

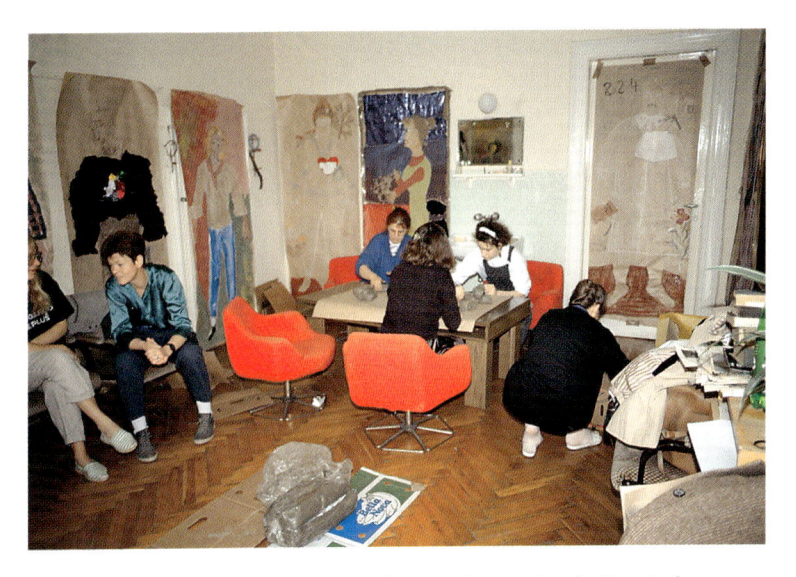

Using family therapy room as workshop, Semmelweis Hospital, Budapest
Photo: Dan Lumley

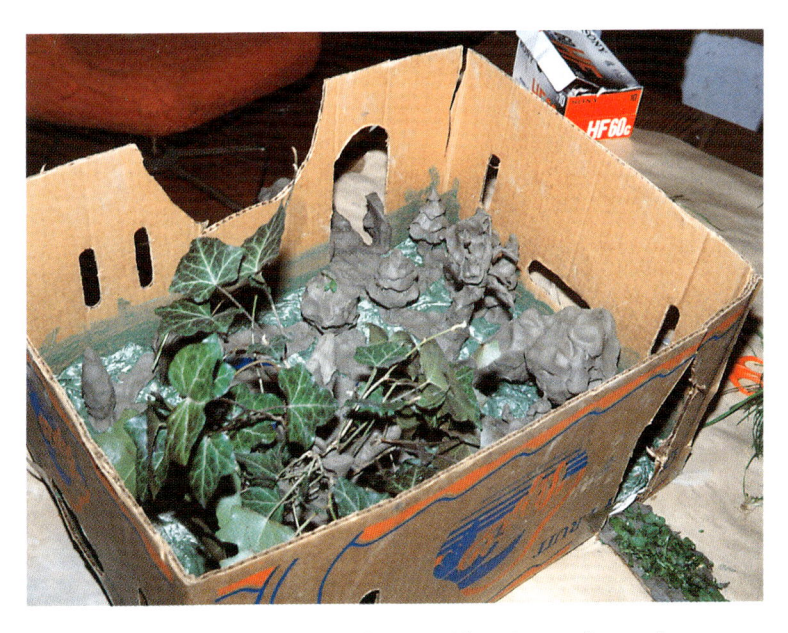

'A "safe space" bringing in outside to inside'. Group clay sculpture, Semmelweis Hospital, Budapest
Photo: Dan Lumley

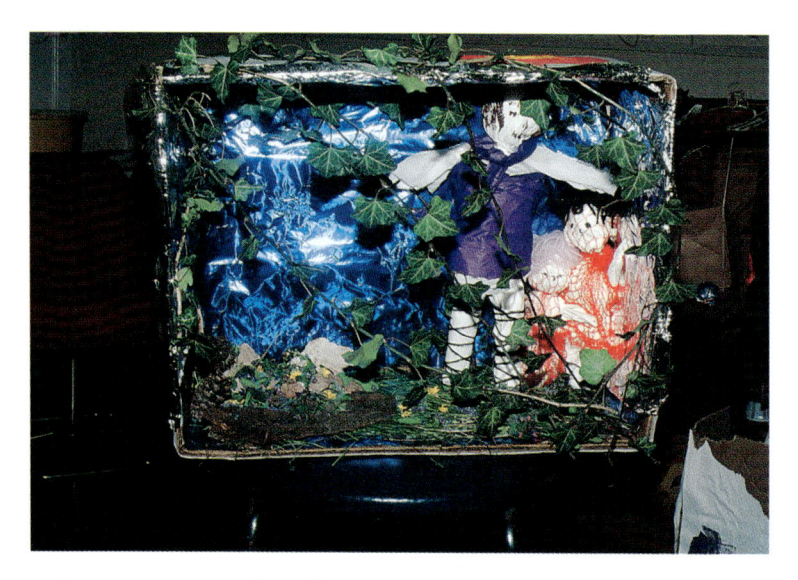

'A box representing the self'. Semmelweis Hospital, Budapest
Photo: Dan Lumley

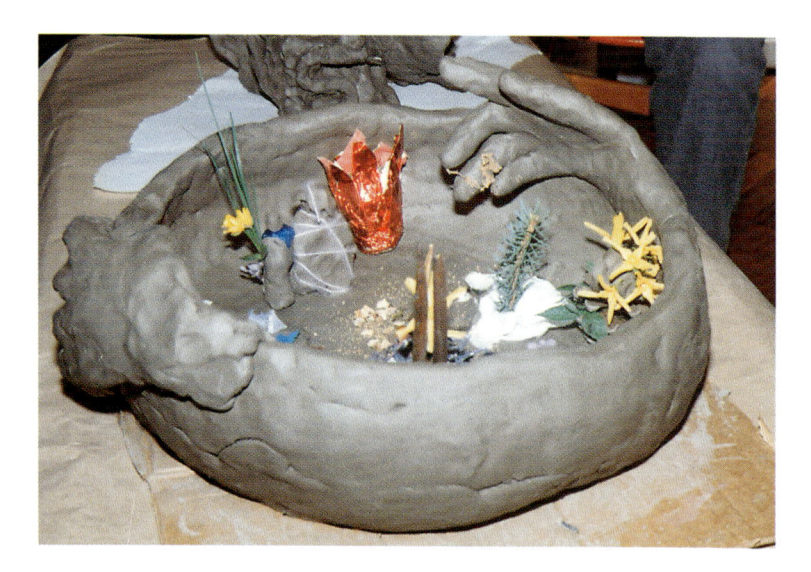

'Bowl of life'. Semmelweis Hospital, Budapest
Photo: Dan Lumley

therapy can be seen as an adjunct to a number of professional activities, such as psychiatry or nursing. Other definitions are 'creative therapy' used in Holland and 'expressive therapy' in France and 'cultural therapy' in Poland, but many countries have adopted a version of 'art' therapy (for example Bulgaria, former Yugoslavia and Russia).

Initiatives such as ECARTE and EABONATA (the European association for professional art therapy organizations) are valuable in beginning dialogue with art therapists, art therapy educators and champions of the process in Europe. What is now fundamentally important to establish is exactly how art therapy is being understood. It will not be possible to do this by seeking definitions from government bodies (even in the UK, where art therapy is regulated, the 'official' definition was way out of date). During the course of the research for this book, I made an attempt but it was totally unsuccessful and produced no definitions at all from government bodies.

Some of the definitions that I did come across in the course of travelling and asking questions have been quite startling and certainly confirm the view of Truss Wertheim in her ECARTE paper. Is it really possible, after all, for a profession to embrace processes so different in kind from making and painting ceramic objects for the tourist market in a craft workshop run by a nursing assistant and working through deep trauma by painting in the presence of an art therapist with several years' experience of training and personal therapy? Both these examples were labelled art therapy. I am not attempting to establish a hierarchy, here by the way, because both could be equally important to a patient. I am simply trying to point out that if the dominant model is the craft-activity one, then the training would no doubt be very different from the latter example. For the patient's sake, we need to be clear about what we are offering in the name of treatment.

In the context of the European Directives, which are discussed below, what if art therapy were to be regulated as in example 1, and an applicant wished to work in Britain, or Holland, where example 2 predominates? What kind of aptitude test or period of adaptation could be offered in this case? Or let us reverse the situation: how could the art therapist in example 2 adapt themselves to the role in example 1?

Art therapists are able to say that art therapy is not art education, nor is it occupational therapy, nor an adjunct to verbal psychotherapy or a diagnostic tool to be used by psychiatrists. Because art therapy has evolved in specific ways, it may not be possible for a similar phenomenon to that, say, of the UK to develop in countries that have not shared a similar social history. It may be that art therapy is so culturally specific that it will be hard, if not impossible, to transfer its concepts and practitioners in the manner demanded by the Directive unless we focus on the social, political and legal context first of all.

The European Directive on the free movement of professionals

In Chapter 1 I referred to the Leeds Conference where a number of professionals gathered to explore the implications of the General Directive for the mutual recognition of qualifications, 89/48. It became clear that there were many concerns among British professionals about the way they could relate to a model of profession that was very different from their own. Neale (1994: 3) pointed out that:

> it is clear that professions as distinct groups have developed rather differently in each member state. History, cultural and economic factors have promoted some occupations to an elite standing in some countries but not others.

She notes that the 1957 Treaty of Rome promised that economic union would mean that community nationals could have the right to work anywhere in the Union and that:

> The Single European Act prompted a flurry of activity to finally achieving this economic free market, and the subsequent legislation certainly challenged the resources of many professional institutions.
>
> (1994: 3)

Some professions began to tackle the issues very promptly and set up committees to deal with European matters, working towards European codes of ethics and practice, standardizing (for example, psychologists) and even influencing legislation where it affects their members (such as engineers). Others have decided that Europe is fairly low on their agenda. The terms of the first directive required there to be competent bodies in each member state to evaluate the qualifications of migrants. Neale mentions that the health professions have most frequently researched differences in professional practice between states and have produced useful publications (1994: 10).

So how does this affect arts therapists? Prior to the British state registration of arts therapists in March 1997, the Council for Professions Supplementary to Medicine (CPSM) was the designated authority on behalf of art, music and dramatherapists. Each of the boards operating under the CPSM was the designated authority for that profession, for example, physiotherapy, occupational therapy, radiography. Once the Federal Board of Arts Therapists is established, the responsibility will fall on its shoulders. The Directives are not intended to influence member states' policy decisions on education and health, but they do forbid a member state making a European National requalify for a profession in order to protect the labour market in any one country. Peter Burley, Deputy Registrar at the CPSM, offered a useful summary of the role of the designated authority (DA) in operating the Directive. He pointed out that the DA would need to be sure that the applicant was actually a practitioner of the profession claimed and that this could be a problem, for there was no guarantee that curricula in different countries overlapped. For instance, someone might call themselves a chiropodist but share very few skills with a UK chiropodist. There were also bona fide professions with competent, properly trained professional practitioners, but they did not correlate with structures and practices in the UK. Another task was to insure that the migrant was genuine, and that they did have a qualification – that is, a diploma as defined by the Directive and issued by a competent authority, which would be the equivalent of a university or institute of higher education. The DA could reject outright anyone whose qualification fell outside the Directive, but conversely had to recognize any falling within it. Burley gives an example of occupational therapy (OT) in the Netherlands, which is taught for four years leading to the professional qualification and three leading to the 'helper' one. Sometimes Dutch helpers sought recognition in the UK, arguing they had had a three year higher education training and quoting the Directive. They were rejected because: (a) they were not OTs because their home national authorities did not define them as such; (b) they were not genuine migrants because they seemed to be trying to play the UK system off against the Dutch; (c) their diploma is not a higher education one and does not correlate to the relevant UK professional curriculum (Burley 1994: 33–4).

One can see from Burley's paper, and from others in the conference proceedings, how complicated it is for well established and large professions to deal with the Directives. To take the example now of a small UK profession (less than 400 members in 1994) we can see how difficult it is for such a small group to act as a competent authority without the backing of an umbrella organization like CPSM. Lydia Tischler, who was then the European secretary for the Association of Child Psychotherapists (ACP), tells us:

> As child and adolescent psychotherapists, the UK is perhaps in a slightly better position than colleagues in Europe, in that the profession is at least recognised in the Health Service. This came to light when, in order to establish the position of the profession in other EC countries, the Association contacted the relevant National Co-ordinators of EC member countries. In most of them child and adolescent psychotherapy (CAPT) is not recognised as a profession and therefore not regulated. This applies to Portugal, Ireland, France, Spain, Denmark and Belgium. In Luxembourg, only those with medical qualifications can practice psychotherapy and that without requiring to undertake further training of any kind . . . in France, psychotherapy can be practised by psychologists whose profession is recognised, but there is no mention of child and adolescent psychotherapy as such. Italy has recently brought in legislation which makes it mandatory to obtain specialist training of at least four years' duration at a university medical school . . . the situation is yet again different in the Netherlands, where CAPT is not a specifically regulated profession but is considered as a specialty of psychotherapy. The only country with recognised training in child-psychotherapy and where child and adolescent psychotherapists can practise within their health service is Germany, but there

they can only do so under the aegis of the medical profession
... psychotherapy is a ubiquitous title which anyone can
claim, whether or not they have training, but also refers to
professionals with widely differing approaches and training
standards.

(Tischler 1994: 121–2)

Tischler describes some of the actions taken by ACP in co-operation with other psychoanalytic psychotherapists to bring together organizations within the mental health field in the public sector in Europe. Over the two years between the establishment of the European Umbrella Organization which had three sections: child and adolescent, adult (individual) and group psychotherapy, considerable progress had been made in, for example, improving training standards, holding scientific meetings and conferences and planning research. Working together with other psychoanalytic psychotherapists was essential, although the ACP retained its own professional identity.

There are many similarities between the issues faced by child psychotherapists and art therapists: both have achieved training standards as a result of much struggle and hard work, and in the case of art therapy these are firmly rooted in the university system. Some advances have been made in establishing similar training within Europe, but there is still a long way to go. Tischler (1994: 125) points out:

However encouraging such progress is, there are differences between the training standards and requirements of the different countries, which have to be heeded.

This creates a dilemma for the profession: how to allow for differences without lowering standards to an extent that sacrifices the quality of work, or where the differences imperceptibly change the boundaries of the profession. This may be peculiar to a profession where the clinical technique relies on the human factor. It is a delicate balance with no easy and quick solutions.

Tischler goes on to address the difficulties of assessing equivalence, pointing out that the really difficult problem as far as child psychotherapy is concerned, is the differences between the personal psychotherapy requirements of each training. It would be hard to see how this shortfall could be made up as normally this goes on parallel with the theoretical and clinical aspects of training. It is one area which the new British Arts Therapy Board, as the competent authority, will no doubt have to deal with sooner or later, since personal therapy is also mandatory in most UK arts therapy training.

Clearly, given the kind of assessment of an applicant's potential for working as an art therapist that is going to be required under the Directive, it is necessary to be precise about the nature and level of the work to be undertaken. In a new profession such as art therapy, the position is far from clear, given the kinds of debates I mentioned above. After all, in most countries in Europe, a visit to a chiropodist would result in a similar process being carried out in each country, or to a physiotherapist – although there might be some slight differences in techniques. It is far from certain that this would be the case for art therapy. One of the criteria to be met in an application for state registration is that the profession has 'a body of knowledge which can be assessed'. Given that art therapy is established as an academic discipline in Britain to Master's level, it was possible to present evidence that there was in fact such a body of knowledge. However, educators are still grappling with the question: what is the body of knowledge which could be said to apply to art therapy and who decides what it is?

Bearing in mind the steps taken by child psychotherapists in contacting European colleagues, we can see that a similar process is underway for arts therapists, beginning around 1990. In an introductory paper to a conference entitled 'Arts therapies education: Our European future' held at St. Albans in 1990, Evans and Dubowski stated that, as far as the European Directive was concerned, the main concerns facing the professions were the nature, length and styles of training in the arts therapies; the question and development of professionalism; the moves towards the concept of closed professions; state and eventually European recognition; the effect of European Community legislation on professional recognition; these processes and the need to develop 'harmonization' within Europe. All were necessary to consider in 'the process of movement towards a profession(s) of Arts Therapies that has a European standard of training with the free movement of professionals throughout Europe' (1991: 4).[1]

One way of beginning to address these two key notions was to have a forum where representatives from colleges already offering a training which conformed to the Directive could meet and discuss their programmes. The European Consortium of Art Therapy Educators (ECARTE) was founded in Nijmegen, Netherlands in 1991 initially by University Rene Descartes, Paris; University of Munster, Germany; University of Aalborg, Denmark; University of Hertfordshire (then Hertfordshire College of Art and Design), St Albans; Hogenschools of Nijmegen, Sittard and Midden Netherlands. Of these founders, only one (Hertfordshire) had training in art therapy at postgraduate level. The programmes in Holland were above the level of a BA Hons in the form of a Higher National Diploma but not at the level of the UK Postgraduate Diploma. The consortium opened its doors to all colleges with an 'approved' programme in any one of the arts therapies as full members, and offered associate status to colleges aspiring to develop training. It was clearly important to have an arena where arts therapy educators could meet and begin to address the key issues of harmonization and equivalence. The task should not, however, be underestimated.

ECARTE is a consortium of universities and higher education institutions working to provide nationally validated and professionally recognized courses in the arts therapies – art, dance, drama and music therapy – within Europe. Its work includes: creating stronger European links in the arts therapies through the international exchange of staff and students; promoting research into methods of art therapy practice within a European dimension; developing opportunities for international study; promoting recognition of qualifications in the arts therapies at European level; ensuring that appropriate and academically sound programmes are provided and maintained. The consortium has reached, as its chair Line Kossolapow (ECARTE 1995: 8) puts it:

> the second stage of the emotional development of ECARTE, the *stage of disenchantment*. For turning an idea from the possible to the actual shows how simple and clear the idea seemed to be and how complex and bewildering the reality is.

This statement seems to echo the view of those concerned with operating the European Directives on the free movement of professionals across Europe.

Note

1 'Harmonization' and 'equivalence' were key words in the Sectoral and General Directives respectively. The General Directive covers professions where entry and employment are regulated by some legally enforceable arrangements and which in the UK would be referred to as 'graduate entry'.

5

Ownership and regulation

When I first began to study art therapy as a profession, I had a layperson's view of profession as something static, or like a person. The idea of a profession going through stages of birth, latency, adolescence and maturity (and eventual death) seemed logical. My perception of profession in this way was possibly influenced by the 'functionalist' theory of professions which predominated until the late 1960s, and was a central influence in the formation of the Act of Professions Supplementary to Medicine (1961) under which arts therapists are now regulated. Along with other officers of the British Association of Art Therapists (BAAT) in 1979, we had studied the requirements for applying for registration under the Council for Professions Supplementary to Medicine (CPSM) but did not feel it was an appropriate body at that time, due to a distrust of the so-called 'medical model' among arts therapists. It was also a fact that there were too few art therapists to constitute a sole professional Board. The concept of 'maturity' was used as one of the criteria to be met for registration (and still is). However, thanks to my PhD supervisor, Dr Barry Cooper, a sociologist and mathematician, I was introduced to the work of American sociologists Bucher and Strauss who offered an alternative to the functionalist model of profession that supported the developmental model I had in mind. They challenged the view of profession as a relatively homogeneous community with shared definitions of role, interests, identity and values, and one that could reach a state of 'maturity' and offered a 'process' model that took into account the dynamic role of conflicts of interest within a profession and the ever-shifting nature of such an entity. In their article 'Professions in process' (1961) they point out that within functionalism there is some room for variation but, by and large, this it is a static view that perceives conflict as negative and threatening to destroy the group itself, rather than as a living, positive contribution to its development. The 'deterministic' character of functionalism, then, leads to a view of civilization in which some groups strive for the 'maturity' that others are assumed to have acquired.

The definition of the term 'profession' has posed many problems for sociologists. Many authors have made suggestions and perhaps one of the most succinct and reflecting of the functionalist position was given by Carr-Saunders and Wilson: 'The application of an intellectual technique to the ordinary business of life, acquired as the result of prolonged and specialised training, is the chief distinguishing characteristic of the profession' (1933: 491). They further suggested that professions were one of the most stable elements in society, in that they formed a resistance (along with the family, church and universities) to 'crude forces which threaten steady and peaceful evolution' (1933: 497).

Most writers up until the late 1960s emphasized the 'altruistic' nature of professions, including those who took a 'traits' approach in which the characteristics which were seen to represent an ideal profession, as opposed to an occupational group, were identified. Tyler, for instance, suggested that the two essential characteristics of a profession were the existence of a generally recognized code of ethics supported by a group discipline and the basing of technical operations on general principles rather than rules of thumb or routine skills (1952: 52–62).

Cogan, on the other hand, concluded that no broad acceptance of any authoritative definition had ever been observed (1953: 33–50). Johnson (1972: 22) agreed with this view:

> The definition of what a profession is becomes a matter of pinpointing what these 'crucial characteristics' are. Such models – more or less abstract – abound in the literature. Theoretical statements have been largely restricted to a discussion and exposition of these characteristics. The result has been a

confusion so profound that there is even disagreement about the existence of the confusion.

Macdonald (1995: 1–5) offers a useful critique of the sociology of professions up until the late 1970s. He suggests that for the sake of sociological clarity we should refer to professions as occupations based on advanced, or complex, or esoteric, or arcane knowledge. He pays particular attention to the work of Larson (1977) who in *The Rise of Professionalism* made significant studies of professionalization and radically departed from prevailing functionalist models. She used the term 'the professional project', which 'emphasizes the coherence and consistency' of a particular course of action, even though 'the goals and strategies pursued by a given group are not entirely clear or deliberate for all the members' (Larson 1977: 6, in Macdonald 1995: 10) Larson was influenced by the sociologist Max Weber who, briefly stated, considered that society is to be seen as individuals pursuing their interests and that this activity generates more or less collectively conscious groups, who are the bearers of ideas that legitimate the pursuit of their interests. Professions engage in competition with each other and with other groups in society, up to and including the state. They have a distinctive place in the class system and this is to some extent determined by the structural features of industrial society. The collective actions of these groups are always significant and can usefully be conceptualized as a strategy of social closure (Macdonald 1995: 27–31). Larson described professionalization as: 'an attempt to translate one order of scarce resources – special knowledge and skills – into another – social and economic rewards' (1977: xvii). In a market-based economy, the aspiring professionals have to form themselves into a coherent group, which then begins to standardize and control the dissemination of the knowledge base. Once they can dominate the market in knowledge-based services they can enter into a bargaining position with the state, allowing further standardization and restricted access to their knowledge by controlling entry to training and the curriculum.

Professional power

On the issue of power and professions, Johnson (1972) points out that groups may see professionalism as a way of gaining autonomy and power to control their own practice for reasons both of increased status and improved service to clients, and that professionalism is a 'successful ideology'. The term is used by many occupational groups who compete for status and income.

Not only do professional groups engage in competition, which generates conflict with others, but they also contain conflict within themselves. Bucher and Strauss's model takes this into account; it is a dynamic one that develops the idea of professions as 'loose amalgamations of segments pursuing different objectives in different manners and more or less delicately held together under a common name at a particular period in history' (1961: 326). In this model a profession is seen in terms of segments, missions and evolution, and in relationship to the political and economic fluctuations of a given society. The segments develop distinct identities and it is the competition and conflict of segments that causes the organization of the profession to shift. This is a particularly useful model to apply to the development of art therapy where conflicts of personal, institutional and state interests caused major shifts of thinking and action (such as the rehabilitation movements necessary after the Second World War, the formation of NHS Trusts and the European Directives which moved art therapists in the UK closer to the Council for Professions Supplementary to Medicine and subsequently state registration, albeit under an Act that currently encompasses the notion of 'maturity') in which art, music and dramatherapists have come together under a single Federal Board. I have described how this process worked in the case of art therapy in the UK up until 1982 in *Becoming a Profession* (Waller 1991) but we can apply it to all professions.

Pauline Neale discusses some features of a profession and its role in society in her introduction to *Creating European Professionals*, the publication resulting from the Leeds Conference:

> Society is looking for people who can be trusted to respect the privilege they have been given, by concentrating on maintaining that privilege on behalf of their group, by accepting the definition and delineation they have negotiated with authority, other professions and society at large.
>
> The existence of a profession depends on the success of a group of practitioners to persuade the state that their particular knowledge base should be restricted, through education,

organisation and regulation, to their own members. Professionalisation may be achieved in a variety of ways, but it is not static, it is an ongoing political process. Professions are viewed by government as interest groups of experts with whom they have an uneasy relationship and indeed the autonomy of a profession to control a particular technical field is constantly tested by the state. Orzack (1992) suggests that while these matters have traditionally been assumed to be a matter for individual nations, this is increasingly being challenged and professionals should look to both European and international institutions as having a growing influence on their practice.
(Neale 1994: 1)

This last suggestion by Orzack is an inevitable consequence of the European Directive on the Free Movement of Professionals discussed in the previous chapter.

In order to meet the requirements for registration under the Act of Professions Supplementary to Medicine in the UK, would-be registrants have to demonstrate that they meet criteria which prove they are more than an 'occupational group' and that they have the potential to be harmful to the public (since public protection is the sole reason for registration). These criteria were restated by Lord Benson in a House of Lords Debate on 18 July 1992, when the status of engineers was being discussed and seem to follow the 'traits' model outlined above. Lord Benson pointed out that eight years previous to the debate, his profession – accountancy – set down nine obligations to the public. The British Association for Art Therapists, and subsequently the professional associations for music and dramatherapy in the UK, were able to demonstrate that they met these obligations and hence went on to achieve state registration. This is the pattern which ARAET is attempting to follow in Swiss-Romande (see Chapter 3). In summary Lord Benson's criteria were:

1 the profession must be controlled by a governing body that directs the behaviour of its members and for their part the members have a responsibility to subordinate their own interests to support the governing body;
2 the governing body must set standards for education and ensure professional competence. Continuing education must also be a requirement;

3 the governing body must set the ethical rules and professional standards to be observed by members, which should be higher than the general law;
4 these rules and standards should be designed for members of the public and not the profession's interest;
5 the governing body must take disciplinary action, including expulsion, if any member fails to observe the rules or is guilty of professional misconduct;
6 work is only reserved for members of the profession by statute so that the public are not at risk of being exploited;
7 practitioners must give information about their experience, competence, capacity to do the work and the fees payable;
8 the members must be independent in thought and outlook, willing to speak their minds without fear or favour, and must not allow themselves to be put under the control or dominance of any person or organization which could impair that independence;
9 in its specific field of learning a profession must give leadership to the public it serves.

Most of the above are now requirements under the PSM Act, except that continuing professional development is not compulsory. It is, though, a strong recommendation of the proposed Health Professionals Act referred to in Chapter 1, which is intended to replace the PSM Act.

Since the Act of Professions Supplementary to Medicine in 1961, only three new professions have been able to join, one of these being arts therapists, as the requirements are so stringent. Many groups seek the title of profession because generally speaking it bestows a positive moral evaluation, and suggests that the work is worthy of esteem in society. It may be viewed as 'an honorific symbol in use in our society' (Becker 1971: 2). Arts therapists in the UK, in seeking to become a state registered profession, have certainly seen this as a way of giving legitimacy to their practice and perhaps enhancing their status, but, as is very clear from Lord Benson's statement and the PSM Act, their first duty has to be to the public and in being a registered practitioner they then submit themselves to stringent rules and codes of conduct under the law. The fact of state registration also means that arts therapists in the UK have now moved into the position described by

Larson (1977), in that the Federal Board of Arts Therapists has the function of controlling access to the profession and exercising control over the training and practice of registrants. However, the market potential of arts therapists will depend upon how successful they are in demonstrating their value to employers and members of the public, and providing evidence of cost-effectiveness. This in turn will depend on how the terms evidence and effectiveness are construed by a cash-strapped National Health Service.

Looking back to the problems outlined by Jacques Stitelmann in Chapter 3, we can see that art therapists in Switzerland are some way from achieving a coherent group status. On the issue of training alone, there are major difficulties to be overcome in that there is relatively little agreement between training institutions on what constitutes an art therapy education, so that to define core standards and competencies would be nearly impossible. In Ireland, on the other hand, work has already progressed, following the formation of the Irish Association and Meitheal, and drawing upon British and American models of training (Chapter 2). Without a clear theoretical, or 'knowledge' base no group can claim to be a profession. Macdonald (1995: 135) comments on this important issue:

> The most important criterion for including an occupation within the scope of this book [on professions] has been that its practice is based on a body of relatively esoteric knowledge. While practice is an essential part of any profession and its training, in the caring professions there is a considerable body of opinion that holds that practice is actually the more important aspect. This is particularly true of nursing, but there and elsewhere this notion has important consequences: first, it devalues the knowledge aspect of the occupation, thus casting doubts on its standing as a profession: and secondly, it emphasizes the caring part of the occupational task, and as caring is something that everyone undertakes in the context of the family, this again devalues the occupation.

British art therapists have been perhaps fortunate (if we look at professionalism as a good thing) in that the founder members of the British Association of Art Therapists, back in the early 1960s, determined that training for art therapy should take place within the university system, thus ensuring that a knowledge base evolved, meeting the criteria of various academic boards and validating bodies, and this was monitored and refined and redefined within the latest set of 'core course' requirements issued by BAAT of 1991. These were an essential element in the bid for state registration. However, the upgrading of training in both clinical and academic aspects, which led to training being extended to two full-time academic years at postgraduate level, did not find immediate favour with the British National Health Service Executive, who accused art therapists of being 'inflationary'. The BAAT pointed out that the only increased costs were to students themselves in that most were self-funding and were prepared to pay for their own training. Arts therapists are currently the only profession registered under the PSM Act who meet the full costs of their training. This gives a certain freedom to the profession to determine a curriculum that is designed to meet the needs of the ever-increasing groups of patients who seek arts therapy, while taking into account the changing needs of the employers. This is a small amount of power, which will be invested in the new Federal Board of Arts Therapists, which will be responsible for approving all programmes in art, drama and music therapy in the UK (around 20 in 1997).

Ownership

From time to time, using Bucher and Strauss's (1961) model, large professions will throw off segments who may then link with other segments from seemingly unrelated groups to form a new specialty. The large professions may wish to lay claim to this new specialty, in other words, to own it. This has happened in Switzerland (see Chapter 3), where art therapy is usually seen as an adjunct to another professional skill and the continuation of this state of affairs prevents a strong knowledge base being built up. Art therapists in the UK have also been subjected to claims of ownership, mainly from occupational therapy (although occasionally from special needs teaching), and in 1977 the Department of Health's Consultative Document on Art, Music and Dramatherapy recommended art therapy should be subsumed under occupational therapy. (Art therapy was referred to by the

Department of Health as a 'linked' profession to occupational therapy for several years). This recommendation was overturned due to a strong campaign in which the support of the Royal College of Psychiatrists and individual Members of Parliament was extremely important. Questions of ownership, and hence others' professional interests have always to be taken into account by a group in process of becoming a profession.

Curiously, ownership of art therapy has never been claimed by artists, possibly because artists do not form a professional group in the UK in the same way as, say, doctors, lawyers, architects or engineers. Yet the art therapy profession is built on the assumption that its entrants have either an initial qualification (first degree) in art or design or demonstrate considerable skill in the theory and practice of art through presentation of a portfolio at interview and continuing artistic development throughout training. We shall see that in many European countries, artists actually reject the concept of art therapy (especially in France and Germany).

The separate identity of art therapy from occupational therapy, having been a source of continuous contention from the 1940s, was eventually warmly supported by the Occupational Therapists Board in 1990, when the application was scrutinized by CPSM in a working party chaired by the Chair of the OT Board, reflecting a major change in attitude since the Consultative Document of 1977. Worth noting is the fact that these professions supplementary to medicine were traditionally 'women's professions' and poorly paid and valued. Having art therapy as part of their remit gave occupational therapists an additional, rather attractive skill to offer and one that could be said to have some roots in the history of the profession, which had included 'arts and crafts'. Moreover, the presence of art therapists in an occupational therapy department enabled the Head Occupational Therapist to receive a higher salary, as grades were based on the 'head count' system.

Given that the professions allied to medicine, except art therapy, were traditionally within schools under the aegis of Departments of Health, moving training for all these groups into the university sector seems to have given greater confidence to the practitioners. This has important gender implications. In the UK the male–female split is about 30–70, with a much greater number of male art therapists in the UK than anywhere else, including the USA.

This might reflect the fact that art therapy training in the UK has always been situated in higher education, that it has not traditionally had a 'handmaiden' connotation, that it has been possible to practise both as an artist and art therapist and that it attracted radical art students from the 1960s who became leaders of the profession. Also, it was linked up with the Trades Union Movement early on and with the 'male' areas of union activity and politics (despite these activities being carried out consistently mainly by the female officers of the British Association of Art Therapists). It is beyond the scope of this book to explore these interesting issues of gender in depth, but necessary to note that in Italy, for instance, there are very few men undertaking art therapy training and it is possible that this has to do with recruitment being from 'care' professions, not traditionally a male stronghold. In the former Eastern Europe, taking the example of Bulgaria, psychiatry and psychology are lower status professions than in the UK and are female-dominated. These professions currently 'own' art therapy, but as an adjunctive element in their work and it is unlikely that a psychiatrist would wish to swap places with an art therapist and other than for personal preference, would have no economic or status-related reasons for doing so.

Regulation

There is much evidence from practitioners all over Europe (that is, according to the number of new associations formed) that they see some form of state (or equivalent recognition) as desirable. However, there are such differences in the social, cultural and legal systems of European countries, and in the way that professions are structured, that the development of art therapy is bound to reflect this.

Taking the example of Italy, where there are now several associations of art therapy, the lack of a common approach and hence of registration can lead to confusion. Mimma della Cagnoletta (pers comm) tells us:

> When I started to talk about art therapy in public in the early 1980s, my major concern was to explain what art therapy was. Nowadays my concern is to explain what art therapy is

not. If in 1980 people would ask 'What is art therapy? What do you do?' Nowadays the same people say 'I have done it', or 'I do it all the time'. Art as a therapeutic tool is used by professionals in the field of psychology and psychiatry. This does not mean they know what they are talking about, or even what they do when they make their patient draw. It only means that it is not as strange or unusual to think that art can be used with mental or physical disabilities, with addiction and so on as it used to be.

Since a growing number of professionals try to use art in their work place, mostly without having a proper training, what comes out is that sometimes the results are less than encouraging and the experiment is left behind and abandoned, closing the door for a well trained art therapist in the future.

The problem we are facing now is of *definition* of a profession that exists but is used in different ways and is taken into consideration at different levels according to who is doing it. A psychiatric nurse may be seen setting up an art studio with psychotics and she will call it art therapy. A psychologist who is also a painter sets up an art studio with patients. A psychiatrist tells an 'operatore' [something like a group worker in England] to start using art with his groups and he will supervise his work and call it art therapy.

Meetings and publications of the European Consortium of Art Therapy Educators (ECARTE) have revealed that within training, there are significant differences across Europe, with some countries having no training at all and others having several, all different, with no co-ordinating association to pull them together. The example of Switzerland (Chapter 3) demonstrates this very clearly. Likewise, the formation of a European group of representatives of professional associations (known as EABONATA) revealed almost irreconcilable approaches to the question of training and professional practice as well as raising a heated debate as to the nature of art itself (see Waller 1992a).

Organizations such as ECARTE and EABONATA try to address similarities and differences and those who join are at least willing to enter a debate. One of the things that art therapists seem prone to do is reinvent the wheel rather than learn from each other. This is reflected also in the literature of English-speaking countries where there is rarely a feeling that, say, the USA and the UK professionals have read each others' work. Perhaps this is something to do with the 'artist' identity within art therapy seeking originality at all costs? The result is that we can waste a lot of time and energy struggling to find ways to do what others have already done, and that we do not pool our knowledge and skills, nor test theory sufficiently. At the stage when art therapists are seeking recognition from universities and government departments, sophisticated strategies need to be adopted that will demonstrate reasonable claims for the profession, take into account the 'interests' of other professions, their possible hostility at worst and indifference at best and the famous 'market economy' that prevails throughout all parts of Europe. For as sure as there are major differences in law, social and cultural factors, education and health care systems, etc. there are likely to be similarities in the way the task can be approached, of ensuring that wherever it can be practised, the work of the art therapist with patients is of the highest standard and is able to be evaluated – and, very importantly, making sure that false claims are not made concerning efficacy in the enthusiasm of pioneering. Then the results of this work can be communicated to all necessary agencies of the country in question, to the general public, the medical and other professions. This is no small task, and if it is to be successful, it needs the united strength of all who are concerned. Many problems lie in this aspect, in that 'ownership' of an idea, a practice, a discipline may be claimed by many people. Territory is established, rival organizations set up and contradictory views are put forward by small groups to government departments who can easily dismiss them out of hand. Such is the trap that the psychotherapists are in danger of falling into and which the United Kingdom Council for Psychotherapy and the British Confederation of Psychotherapists, among other national organizations in the UK, are trying to address. However, ownership of psychotherapy has now been claimed by at least the medical and psychological professions of several European countries. Art therapists in the UK have an Act of Parliament legitimizing them and protecting the public they serve so there is a precedent. It is unlikely that art therapists across Europe will avoid the traps of nationalism and territorialism, and a more realistic and dynamic position is to anticipate conflict and try to deal with it as a necessary part of a developing profession.

In summary, the striving towards professionalism usually comes from the followers who are seeking new work opportunities, within a role that gives a feeling of self-worth and of being valued by one's society. This push is unlikely to come from professionals who have acquired additional skills and who remain in their original role, unless they are driven by personal desire and dissatisfaction with that role. It is unusual for professionals to move from a higher paid and higher status position (for example, doctor) to one of the professions allied to medicine, such as art therapy, although there are a few examples in the UK where the enjoyment of the job has prevailed over other considerations.

This raises important questions for training, especially when the trainees already have a core profession. Are the trainees being socialized into art therapists or are they learning a set of adjunctive skills? I hope this question posed by this book will exercise colleagues engaged in training programmes across Europe.

6

Social and cultural contexts

It is only since the early 1980s in the UK at least that the sociocultural contexts of medicine, particular psychiatry, psychotherapy and art therapy seem to have been seriously discussed. Littlewood and Lipsedge, writing in *Aliens and Alienists* in 1982, drew attention to the seriousness of this omission, which resulted in patients from various ethnic groups failing to be correctly diagnosed, or being more often diagnosed as schizophrenic or psychotic and admitted to acute admissions wards. Very rarely were they referred for psychotherapy, which was not then indicated for these conditions. The cultural context in which any profession develops will undoubtedly influence the knowledge base and the relationship with other professions, with the law and the state. We cannot assume, and indeed evidence shows, that art therapy will have a different professional shape in Britain from, say, in Switzerland, Germany or France. This is one of the many reasons why operation of the European Directives on the free movement of professionals is so complex. Macdonald (1995) usefully addresses issues of historical and cultural context with reference to medicine and law in a chapter 'The cultural context of professions', looking at Britain, the USA, France and Germany. When looking at the development of art therapy in both France and Germany further on in this chapter, it is helpful to bear in mind his comment that:

France and Germany were characterized, at the formative periods for professions, by centralized states, and while the various revolutions that these societies have experienced have changed their political institutions, they have not altered their centralization nor the notion of state responsibility for the public control, and even provision, of knowledge-based services. France differed from Germany in that it threw off its despotism, but the ensuing participation and representation was not of a kind to allow much penetration of the state by civil society. In consequence, knowledge-based services have remained in the ambit of the state, restricting the success of the professional project.

(1995: 97)

Macdonald also makes brief references to the (erstwhile) communist states in which knowledge-based services were provided and regulated entirely by the state. This situation is obviously changing but the influence will still be felt, as we shall see in discussion of the Czech and Slovak republics. The sociocultural context has to be taken into account when considering the growth of ideas and the knowledge base of a profession.

In any discipline, ideas have been in circulation for some time, but at certain points in history they get taken up, spread and a new discipline develops (see Waller 1991). Taking Britain as an example, in the 1940s the return of so many wounded servicemen from the Second World War gave impetus to a new range of rehabilitation programmes, many of which were staffed by artists and craftspeople. Occupational therapy and group psychotherapy also had their origins in this period. It was a time of hope and renewal, following the catastrophic events of both world wars, which left their effects deeply imprinted on the physical and mental state of all those concerned. It was at this point that Adrian Hill began his pioneering work, and being a man who deeply believed in the principle that art is for all he organized a campaign to spread the notion of the healing value of art throughout sanatoria and eventually psychiatric hospitals in the 1940s. Others were working at the same time and came together under the auspices of the National Association for Mental Health which progressed the ideas during the 1950s, eventually leading to the formation of the British Association of Art Therapists in 1964

(Waller 1991). British Art Education, the liberal 'child art' movement and popularity of art classes among the general public, together with British pragmatism were some of the influencing factors. Art therapy thus developed with a comparator of art teaching, or adult education lecturing while at the same time doctors, psychiatrists and in particular Jungian analysts were sometimes encouraging their patients to make art that was subsequently used in diagnosis or in psychotherapy sessions. Art therapy in the UK has always been a grass roots movement, from its earliest days linked up with the Trades Union Movement, first with the National Union of Teachers and later with a large Health Service Union, which has recruited from art and design graduates who tended to be among the more radical or divergent thinkers of our society.

Art education in Britain during the 1960s began to be influenced by the 'basic design' concepts stemming from the Bauhaus movement, which began in the Weimar republic, was subject to persecution by the Nazis due to the left-wing radicalism of its teachers, moved to Dessau, Berlin and finally dispersed to Chicago where its influence continued to permeate art and architecture education. Some elements of the Bauhaus ideology could be said to have appeared in British art therapy education, with its emphasis on the dynamics of form and experiential workshops.

The 'down to earthness' of the founder art therapists was, though, sometimes tempered by a kind of romanticism or sentimentalizing of artistic activity, to be found among medical colleagues and art therapists concerning notions such as the 'mad genius' or that art is inherently 'good for people' in the sense of improving their minds. Generally speaking though, artists who worked in hospitals during the 1950s onwards were driven by a sense of outrage at the lack of opportunity for communication, and the poor quality of life of patients in the old Victorian psychiatric hospitals. Many of the pioneers of art therapy in the UK spoke of getting into art therapy 'accidentally' through being asked to teach an art class in a hospital or patients' club but then becoming totally caught up by the need of the patients for some form of creative expression. This work offered a more meaningful and satisfying role to many artists than art teaching per se or the other major occupation for art graduates at that time, commercial art (see Waller 1991).

From as far back as the early 1960s, art therapy was conceived by the British Association of Art Therapists as an autonomous occupational group and later (1981) after some considerable efforts in public relations and campaigning by BAAT, became regulated in the National Health Service with terms and conditions of service, and salaries, equivalent to those of occupational therapists, physiotherapists and dieticians. The line from this position to state registration was not without its hitches, but on the whole things progressed fairly logically in Larson's (1977) terms as a 'professional project' with increasing refinement in entry to training and curriculum design. The regulation of 1981 was followed by approval of postgraduate art therapy training by the National Joint Council, the body which approves qualifications for social services professions. These events gave British art therapists confidence to begin to examine their discipline in depth and publications from well-known and respected publishing houses started to appear, many of which focused on case material or sketched out theoretical frameworks.

The 1980s, with the aggressive market economy philosophy, and move towards the privatization of health and reorganization into trusts, saw an end to collective bargaining by the trades unions, and the rather cumbersome but useful machinery for determining salaries at a national level, the Whitley Council, began to be disbanded. A Pay Review Body, which also covered nurses and midwives, was established and reported annually. The post-modern fragmentation of British society was well underway, with Margaret Thatcher's famous words: 'There is no such thing as society'. Nevertheless, art therapists remained firmly in contact with their union colleagues, and still insisted on all registered members being members of a recognized trades union. This requirement was reaffirmed at an AGM and still exists. However, to be state registered, but not a member of BAAT, there is no such requirement. A qualified person can simply go on the register. Whatever issues will emerge from the existence of a new Federal Board of arts therapists in its relationship with BAAT, the profession is firmly established.

Clearly, from meetings of ECARTE, EABONATA, articles in journals and from the contributors to this book, this is not the situation elsewhere. Each country has its own cultural, social, legal and philosophical context out of which art therapy will either develop or not, as the case may be. It is important to look at the historical context, in terms of influences from other fields, such as psychoanalysis, art education, aesthetics, sociology. Several contributors have managed to trace the links. Let us look, for example, at Vera Vasarhelyi's account of the development of early psychoanalytical thinking in Hungary:

> Among Freud's closest and earliest co-workers were a number of Hungarian analysts, just as there were among his later followers and disciples: Sandor Ferenczy, Mihaly Balint, Geza Roheim and Imre Hermann – just to mention a few. Melanie Klein's Hungarian connection is also well known. In the 1910s, the Hungarian capital, Budapest, together with Vienna, was in the fore-front of psychoanalysis. After the 1919 revolution there, the first Chair in psychoanalysis was established, albeit only for a short time. However, historical developments destroyed this process for most of the century. During the racial intolerance of the 1920s and 30s (almost all analysts were Jewish) psychoanalysis retreated into a form of internal exile – similar to that of the 1950s, 60s and 70s. However, psychoanalysis survived, and despite decades of a forced loyalty by psychiatrists to Pavlovian Neurology, never stopped being practised secretly.
>
> In order to fully understand the resilience of the profession, it is necessary to describe the early development of ideas and clinical practice, which in my view was instrumental for the survival of the profession in a hostile environment. It seems to me important to clarify that only psychiatrists and psychologists were allowed to train and practice as analysts and psychotherapists. As this is still so today, this model decided the question of eligibility for training on the Postgraduate Visual Psychotherapy Course.
>
> The Hungarian school of psychoanalysis had – despite their close alliance with Freud – soon developed an independent voice. Sandor Ferenczy – an outstanding clinician – developed his own analytical technique and proposed a new method, that of the 'mutual analysis'. This was a crucial departure from the classical assumption of the neutrality of the analyst, since it fundamentally changed the analytical relationship from a strictly authoritarian one to an egalitarian

one. Ferenczy described with unprecedented honesty how a patient was able to help him with his own unresolved feelings at a stage when the analysis seemed to have come to a dead end. He felt that his mentor, Freud, as well as his peers, did not wish to humanise psychoanalysis and were unwilling to look at any form of professional hypocrisy. His innovations seemed to threaten the establishment and his position increasingly became that of an outsider and heretic within the analytical community. He was declared 'insane' by them: an interesting parallel with methods of dealing with dissidents by another totalitarian establishment in the former Soviet Union. Ferenczy in his recently published clinical diary described a desperate wish to regain Freud's approval and understanding of his innovations and ideas. His clinical diary, which he finished just before his death in 1932, was suppressed until 1988 by the psychoanalytical community.

It was not only Ferenczy who diverted from the established 'party line' of Freud and the International Association. Imre Hermann questioned the validity of the theory of female penis envy on the basis of his own clinical findings as early as the 1920s. His understanding of the female's wish for the penis was in the context of object relations – the penis as a desirable, good object to be internalised – and not within the context of penis envy and feelings of inferiority. The logical consequence was that he questioned the validity of the castration complex as well as the assumption of the passivity of female sexuality. Hermann not only reviewed some of the basic tenets of analytical thinking but also contributed ideas that were far ahead of his time. In the 1920s he developed his theory of attachment and separation, in which he compared biological processes with processes of the unconscious instincts within the individual. He introduced the importance of early attachment between mother and baby and therefore rearranged the accepted sequence in the psychological development of the human infant. The consequence of his assumption was that he believed that the infant starts as part of a dyadic unit and not as an individual who learns only later to form relationships and be ready to socialise. His findings were very similar to ideas developed much later by Bowlby in Great Britain.

> The innate strength and courage of the Budapest School came from its history of independent thought, the willingness to put what they felt was the truth above political compromise, and the ability to survive in a hostile external environment.
>
> (Vasarhelyi personal communication)

It is clear from Vera Vasarhelyi's description that in Hungary she had a complex series of cultural issues to take into account, not the least being the interruption of a process of psychological thought during the post-war period in Hungary and the major change brought about by the shift towards western Europe in the early 1990s. Nevertheless, Hungary shared with other European countries the view that artists do not/should not become therapists and that this occupation should be reserved for medical specialists.

In a neighbouring country, Austria, which was for so long linked with Hungary during the period of the Austro-Hungarian Empire, we find many similarities but the development of art therapy has part of its roots in art education, as in Britain. Wolfgang Mastnak (personal communication) writes:

> The sources of recent art therapy in Austria are to be found in various art theories of education of the 1920s and 30s. These trends stressed creative expression, unconventional sensitive experience, and an open consciousness of the arts. This development influenced therapeutic pedagogy as well. Although it is not possible to fix a distinct date of the beginning of art therapy in Austria, the foundation of the 'Deutschsprachige Gesellschaft fur Psychopathologie und Ausdruck', DGPA (German-speaking Society for Psychopathology and Expression) in 1969 in Linz (Upper-Austria) played an important role within the development of art therapy in Austria. From 1971 to 1985 this society was directed by Wolfgang Mueller-Thalheim, psychiatrist and neurologist, who fostered investigations on interdependence between psychopathology of expression and art therapy (*Ausdruckspsychologie und Kunsttherapie*) and who was the first to teach this special field as a university subject in Austria.

Alfons Reiter, psychoanalyst and professor of clinical psychology at Salzburg University, has played the most outstanding role within Austrian art therapy. He contributed to the scientific establishment of art therapy (Reiter 1978, 1983) and stressed the interdependency of pieces of art and self-images (1982, 1994). A main part of his investigations, however, focused on paintings of depressive patients. A synoptic analysis of both their pathological and artistic phenomena resulted in new art-related methodological, diagnostic, and therapeutic insights (Reiter 1985).

Deriving his scientific research from psychoanalysis, Reiter opened new approaches to the symbolic and metaphoric contents of visual structures. As one of the most important activities of Alfons Reiter we should mention the international congress for art therapy in 1989 in Salzburg. This congress increased the public awareness of art therapy in Austria, involved new international contacts, and progressed the idea of establishing institutionalised training courses for art therapy in Austria.

From about 1985 Mastnak has been developing integrated 'artistic' therapies. Focusing on the interdependence of music therapy, drama therapy, dance therapy and art therapies, he developed an approach called 'polyaesthetic therapy'. Its main ideas were influenced by Wolfgang Roscher's 'polyaesthetic education' (Roscher 1976) and Claus Thomas' applications of Polyaesthetic Education to paediatrics and therapeutic pedagogy. Acting as head of the department of music and body-orientated therapies at the neuropsychiatric hospital in Salzburg, Mastnak advanced his theories and examined them in clinical practice (Mastnak 1994a, b).

He located four different theoretical approaches to art therapy in Austria:

1 Art therapy that derives from classical psychotherapeutic or psychological theory, the most popular approach being based on psychoanalysis or at least closely combined with depth psychology. This form of art therapy emphasizes the symbolic meaning of images and their relationship to the unconsciousness. The most significant representative of this trend is Alfons Reiter but other substantial influences on psychoanalytical art therapy are Rainer Danzinger and Helmut Paulus (1995).
2 Art therapy that mainly derives from artistic practice and the science of art. This is a multidimensional approach that incorporates

anthropological aspects, artistic experiences, self-reflection, and clinical analysis.
3 An integrative approach to art therapy that seems to be gaining importance. 'Polyaesthetic therapy' (Mastnak 1994a, b) is the most practised and most regarded therapy of this kind in Austria. It combines music, drama, dance, and art with body work, classical and alternative therapeutic concepts. The arts not only serve as a therapeutic medium, but as a meaningful way to carry on one's life. Therapeutic work by means of the arts helps to reactivate essential creativity, and artistic work helps to get rid of neurotic fixations, and to stabilize cognitive, volitional, and emotional human functions.
4 'Individualistic' art therapies are influenced by personal experiences, intuition and the reflections of the therapist. This type of art therapy is practised privately or at hospitals, where art therapists mostly justify their methods by virtue of their long clinical experience. Efficient practice may result in publications of the most successful clinical cases and their leading ideas. Nevertheless, there is no common and consistent theory.

The work of Berta Klement, a pioneer of the arts therapies in Austria, may be placed here. A staunch supporter of international meetings and an enthusiastic networker, Berta Klement has set up a self-help group called 'Music Workshop' (*Musische Arbeitsgemeinschaft*) and is dedicated to the statement: 'Art helps healing' (*Kunst Hilft Heilen*), and to the integrative value of engaging in the practice of visual and musical arts. She is part of a tradition of workers – including the social psychiatrist Joshua Bierer, who set up art clubs for patients in the UK in the 1940s and 50s – who have established settings where current or ex-patients may go to learn to paint, or indeed to continue their professional work in the arts fields.

Moving to the Czech Republic and Slovakia, which were previously in eastern European bloc and hence philosophically influenced by Marxism and dialectic materialism, though also by the Austro-Hungarian empire, we find that art therapy is developing, but is dependent on certain individuals working in isolation. Martin Bojar, in 1992 Minister of Health of the Czech Republic, wrote that the Czech health care system was in a difficult state due to the profound changes that had occurred in that country.

The aim was to reform the system, to create a democratized health care system that combined public, private and state sectors, which was a completely new phenomenon in the Czech Republic. He stressed the importance of community based models, and the need for financing the reforms through health insurance schemes (Bojar 1993: 4–5). Within such a major upheaval, art therapy has a difficult job to establish itself. Wolfgang Mastnak (personal communication) writes:

> Some recent interviews in the Czech Republic showed that psychiatry and psychotherapy mainly ignored humanistic psychology and alternative approaches during the communist era.
>
> Nevertheless, there were some isolated attempts to cope with the materialistic restrictions. Due to the scientific and clinical interest of Dr Cimicky, head physician at the psychiatric hospital in Bohnice, Prague, one of these attempts resulted in the incorporation of artistic activities into psychiatric treatment.
>
> The outstanding role in Czech art therapy, however, is played by Dr Milan Kyzour in Kaplice. For decades he has practised, taught and organised art therapy in South Bohemia, namely at the University of Budweis [Bratislava]. In Kyzour's method, images are produced within a group therapy session. Subsequently they are analysed either within the group or alone with the patient. Kyzour's method was influenced by depth psychology, namely by C.G. Jung's theory of the archetypes, focuses on the symbolic meaning of images and profits from the metaphorical sense of the arts. Diagnosis as well as the therapy itself are closely connected with this method of interpretation. The art therapy training takes four years and the curriculum incorporates various subjects which refer to the interdependence of psychological disorder and artistic intervention, such as, e.g. general psychopathology, individual anamnesis and artistic expression, diagnostic analysis of images, techniques of painting and drawing, special art-therapeutic methods, and history of the arts. The training courses take place on weekends and are designed for psychologists, physicians and other licensed therapists. They are seen as additional qualifications [to a core profession].

Art therapy following Kyzour's method is designed to be practised at educational institutions, welfare centres, health care centres, centres of social rehabilitation, and charities. The Budweis [Bratislava] department of art therapy is fully accepted by the University Institute of Psychotherapy in Prague.

In Slovakia, the development of art therapy has been slow, and follows behind music therapy. Wolfgang Mastnak and Klaudia Kosalova (personal communication) explain:

Slovakia is situated to the east of Austria, to the south of Poland, and to the north of Hungary. It often gets confused with Slovenia, the most western country of the former Yugoslavia. Although both countries belong to the Slavic speech area, Slovakia and Slovenia have different languages and a different culture.

Art therapy in Slovakia is neither widely practised nor does it play an important role within the national health care system. No institution or organisation is specifically concerned with art therapy. Nevertheless there are various therapeutic activities in Slovakia which are neither popular nor centrally registered. During the communist regime, the official philosophy was based on materialism. By that means therapy was mainly connected with biological methods or empirically measurable interventions like behavioural approaches. The common standard of [psycho]therapy was not compatible with the idea of aesthetic therapies. Scientific paradigms changed together with the official end of the communistic era. The new philosophic, social, and clinical situation leads us to expect both scientific and practical advance of art therapy. This might result in an adequate acceptance of art therapy by the Slovakian authorities.

When considering the influences from various disciplines on the development of art therapy, it is clear that the International Society, known as SIPE and referred to in Chapter 3, has been instrumental in drawing the attention of psychiatrists to the therapeutic, or perhaps rather more, diagnostic potential of art. The society is based at St Anne's Hospital in Paris, where there is also a centre of the same name, founded by Professor Robert Volmat in 1954. It hosts many seminars and annual conferences throughout the world. At the conference in Biarritz, 1997, it was proposed to change the name to psychopathology of expression *and* art therapy, marking a major change in the orientation of the society. The origins of the Society for the Psychopathology of Expression (SIPE) were in the first world congress of psychiatry, held in Paris in 1950. An exhibition of patients' art work was shown in St Anne's Hospital, the Sorbonne University and a health centre in Charenton, consisting of about 2000 art works by 350 patients from 16 different countries. This exhibition formed the basis of a thesis by R. Volmat, entitled 'L'art psychopathologique', which was published in 1956. Volmat's thesis made a relationship between the symbols and themes in the art work and so-called 'primitive' art, as well as with twentieth-century art. He also tentatively suggested that the art work could be used for analytic or therapeutic purposes. Influenced by this study, Jean Delay proposed an international society for the psychopathology of expression at the Verona psychiatry congress in 1959, where the first International Symposium of Art and Psychopathology also took place. A national society, the Societé Française was founded in 1964. There are now branches of SIPE in most countries, including one in Scotland that was founded in the early 1960s and quietly flourished, though with few members, due to the enthusiasm of the late Professor Ralph Pickford and Joyce Laing, both founder members of BAAT. SIPE emerged as a result of interest by doctors in the graphic expression of patients in psychiatric hospitals at the end of the nineteenth century.

Geoff Troll, an English art therapist who lives and works in France, and who until 1995 was President of the French Association of Art Therapists (which has no connection with SIPE), writes:

> In 1872, a French doctor published a text about paintings by the insane, *Etude médico-légale sur la folie*. In this text André Tardieu developed the myth of the mad artist. Thirty-five years later Doctor Paul Meunier published *L'art chez des fous* (*Art by Mad People*), a revolutionary book for its time. It was impossible to imagine that a recognized 'serious' psychiatrist could be associated with this sort of concept; in fact, he had to publish under the pseudonym Marcel Reja.
>
> This book was written for the general public and spoke about the spontaneous quality of art work by mentally ill

people, especially their capacity to find a sort of creative innocence – a sort of return to childhood in a wild primitive way. It achieved its aim and attracted the interest of a large public, and especially many artists.

In 1915, Dr A. Marie, Paul Meunier's head doctor, opened a museum in Villejuif consecrated to the art works of psychiatric patients.

Around about the same time as W. Morgenthaler published his first articles about A. Wölfli in Switzerland, and H. Prinzhorn published *Bildnerei der Geisteskranken* in Germany, H. Delacroix (1927) published *Psychologie de l'art* in Paris and Dr Marie organized many exhibitions showing works from within the psychiatric institutions in various Parisian galleries. One of their main objectives was to open the walls of the asylum so that patients' work could be seen in public.

In the early 1940s, the surrealist movement – including Breton – were intrigued by the creation of so-called psychiatric art, which became somewhat the vogue. In 1949 Dubuffet created the Compagnie de l'Art Brut. His main objective was to promote and encourage a movement of art by non-artists, many of whom came from the psychiatric milieu. Many of these works can now be seen in the *collection de l'art brut* in Lausanne.

Professor R. Volmat and Dr C. Wiart devoted many years in the 60s to detailed studies of patients' art work and its documentation. They were probably influenced by the work of Paul Meunier at the beginning of the century, and A. Marie, with their exhibitions of psychopathology. Most of their material is now in the Centre d'Etudes de l'Expression in Paris which has four principle functions: therapy, research, teaching and documentation.

The Centre International de documentation sur les expressions plastiques (CIDEP) was created in 1963 and now has a library of over 4000 reviews, articles and books. They also have an *iconothèque* of about 100,000 paintings and drawings on slides and over 1,500 clinical dossiers. The CIDEP also houses the museum Singer Polignac which organizes permanent exhibitions and several temporary itinerant exhibitions of art psychopathology.

The Societé Française de Psychopathologie de l'Expression was formed in 1964 and is a member of the International association de psychopathologie de l'expression created in 1959 by Professor R. Volmat and Dr. G. Rosolato representing France.[1]

Some influences of SIPE and *art brut* are also found in Germany, and of course in Switzerland, which Jacques Stitelmann discussed in Chapter 3, and Austria where the psychiatrist Leo Navratil founded a house for artist-patients at Gugging.

In Hungary, however, a professor of psychiatry, Istvan Hardi, has tried to bring together art therapy and the psychopathology of expression in several joint conferences, and has sponsored workshops by some British art therapists. This has led to a growing interest in art therapy among Hungarian psychiatrists.

Karin Dannecker (personal communication) discusses the influences of these movements on the development of art therapy in Germany:

> Despite the attempt of some to root art therapy in ancient times (which discipline doesn't?), most colleagues mention that a more concrete beginning of a development towards art therapy can be seen in the liberalization movements in psychiatric medicine during the second half of the last century. At the time when asylums were considered not to be only places where the insane could be kept away from the public, but also where psychological treatment could take place, some progressive psychiatrists made important observations: their patients seemed to be driven by an urge to express themselves using pieces of newspaper, wood and other available materials to draw, to paint, and to create sculptures.
>
> Painting studios were established where these patients could work with simple artist media. The event of Prinzhorn's book *Artistry of the Mentally Ill* in 1922 in Germany, and the following excited reactions of artists like Dubuffet, Klee, Kandinsky, Dali, etc. has offered an opening key argument not only for artists but also for medical people to bring the art of so-called outsiders into a new light. The traditional romantic attitude that mentally disturbed or ill people are the real artist geniuses still prevails in some approaches.

From the 1980s on the acknowledgement of the 'Artists from Gugging', a group of psychiatric patients near Vienna, Adolf Wölfli and other gifted and promoted institutionalized 'outsiders' has fallen on fruitful ground. They reached the public in the form of exhibitions, books and symposia. The major issues in the discussions which evolved were centred around the sensitive relationship between art and therapy. Some argue that the 'raw' psychic material of the mentally ill expressed in pictures, the *Art Brut*, form a basic model for art therapy. But most practitioners report that art therapy rarely encounters the 'gifted' patient. Instead art therapists meet people who cannot use art or other creative material to express and to communicate their thoughts and emotions, and it is their task to enable their patients to develop a capacity for symbolic expression. The dispute about *l'Art Brut* as a cornerstone for art therapy started in the 80s with the first exhibitions of patients' artwork and is still prevailing today.

In 1985 an English branch of SIPE was formed to host the eleventh Triennial Congress. This took place at Goldsmiths College, London, and was jointly hosted by BAAT. Unlike most other previous SIPE conferences, this one was attended by a large number of art therapists from the UK, the rest of Europe and the USA – although others came from South America, Israel and Japan as well. It was at this conference that the difference in approach between those who saw art therapy, or the psychopathology of expression as an adjunct to their primary occupational role (e.g. psychiatry, psychology) and those who saw it as their primary career became very evident. In particular, British and American art therapists were disinclined to discuss art work outside the context of the therapeutic relationship, whereas others might look at paintings from a diagnostic or psychopathological viewpoint. There was a tendency for publications of the *Centre d'Etude de l'Expression* to focus on 'art and madness', and on the psychopathological aspects of creation, which is antipathetic to the position of UK art therapists (for example, see Barthelemy *et al.* 1996, which includes papers on Mozart, Dostoevsky, Hoffmann and Edgar Allan Poe.

In discussing some of the approaches to art therapy in Germany, Karin Dannecker explains how some of them have evolved.

We can see the influence of the SIPE in these developments, which in some cases has led to artists becoming hostile to the 'pathologizing' of art. Karin Dannecker (personal communication) reports having identified three main approaches:

> one relying mainly on art with little emphasis on therapeutic aspects, the second is rooted in psychotherapy and minimizes the artistic processes to serve as a special form of therapy. And the third is the anthroposophic approach, based on the teaching of Rudolf Steiner, as a holistic and spiritual use of art to harmonize an unbalanced life.

She recalls a conference when art therapists from these different approaches came together:

> I remember one of the first art therapy conferences where artists working in hospitals presented their work with patients with great enthusiasm: every move with a brush on the paper was a sign of liberation; the production was idealized and – with no hesitation – perceived as comparable with modern art expression. Questioned about possible therapeutic effects or goals in relation to the treatment by doctors or other therapists, the answer was purposefully negative: any exchange with medical or psychological people would deepen a stigma already put on the patients as sick and pathologically determined people, and it would prevent the growth of uncensored creativity.
>
> Some responsibility for such a radical attitude of separating art from medicine and psychology might be found in the historical encounters which artists have made with psychological theories about art. Early psychoanalytic writings indicated that artists are driven by conflict, using the form of their art to hide unconscious contents. Early psychoanalysts assumed that the artist tries to control instinctual needs and impulses by adapting to outer reality through artistic work. Placing the artist close to the neurotic, the psychoanalytic approach was not really able to convey to artists that it can offer valuable ways of understanding personality and the psychological aspects of creativity.
>
> Unfortunately most of these artists are not familiar with later writings that view the art process and product as a

means to communicate, to react and to grow for every creative personality: as the capacity for symbolic expression that is given only to human beings. This later literature has also not reached the related professions; instead distrustful projections persist about the work of art therapists. As already indicated, the selective and redundant readings of psychoanalytic literature has led some artists to express scepticism about the use of art in the context of therapy. The major argument of artists to whom I have talked in and outside of art academies is still today that art cannot be applied in therapy without losing essential elements of the autonomy of art. There is a great suspicion that art can experience a kind of misuse when introduced into therapy. This happens when the art part in therapy is used and described mainly as a diagnostic tool for medical treatment. The interpretation of pictorial expression by pointing at pathological personality traits creates truly deep mistrust about the seriousness of art therapists. This includes some of the approaches of verbal psychotherapy that make use of pictures as a 'short cut' to the unconscious of the patients. These 'diagnostic' approaches make artists concerned that the most important aspects of art are lost when it is introduced into therapy; they fear that art is reduced to being an additional tool for medically oriented treatment.

Mimma della Cagnoletta (personal communication) confirms the same situation in Italy, when discussing the influences on art therapy there – that is, the indifference or hostility of artists towards art therapy:

If we want to list the major influences on art therapy, we have to take into account different sources:

- psychology of art and psychopathology of expression, through university level studies, through the Society for Non-Verbal Communication, through Lombroso studies (these have influenced the work of most psychiatrists);
- Anglo-Saxon art therapy theory and practice, through the Art Therapy Italiana (ATI) and Associazione per lo Studio del Disagio Giovanile (ADEG) schools, in connection

with which psychoanalytic literature has been extensively studied;
- American and English Object Relations Schools. Winnicott (1971a, b) is the biggest influence and has stimulated interest in art therapy on the part of related professionals such as psychoanalysts and psychotherapists.

The minor influence comes from artists. Even if they have done a lot of work, they have stayed very isolated, denying and despising the influence of psychoanalytic and psychotherapeutic sources on what they are doing, and thus limiting the spread of their work.

The ambivalent attitude of artists towards art therapy is also found in the UK, where the profession is one of the few career options available for art graduates. It seems clear that certain texts in the field of art and psychoanalysis have given artists the impression that visual creativity is linked to neuroticism, or that the art work of patients is dissected in the interests of a crude diagnostic formula, or that only people who are not 'real' artists go into art therapy (or art teaching). Yet the roots of art therapy lie so strongly in the rich world of image, symbol, metaphor and in the rituals and traditions of each culture, that it would be sad if the professionalism of art therapy towards subjects allied to medicine should cause a rift to develop between artists and art therapists.

The roots of art therapy might also be seen as lying in the traditional rituals and practices of rural communities that have largely died out during the twentieth century in Europe. That is to say, involvement in making art objects for a specific communal purpose may have served a useful function in integrating an individual with the group. Jacques Stitelmann (personal communication) suggests that this may have been the case in pre-industrialized Switzerland:

> If one accepts a wide definition of art therapy as an original theory and practice that facilitates the social and psychological integration of people, and that gives them a sense of the uniqueness of their lives and their future by using expressive, creative and artistic mediation, it is interesting to note

that in Switzerland, like elsewhere, individual quests for self-knowledge have been promoted through the interventions of social, religious and mystical groups.

Therapeutic activity has its roots in mythical, ritual, religious and sacred spheres, as well as in social practices that integrate the person into a coherent cultural milieu, which through linking every individual to the group gives meaning to each life. Our museums are full of prehistoric and neolithic objects which have served these integrative aims. They are imbued with a powerful aesthetic.

Switzerland has long been rooted in its farming tradition, nestling in valleys and introspective places, which has ensured that its traditional practices have survived. They have been recorded in 'folklore' since the nineteenth century. By this I mean that these practices are not a really authentic, symbolic part of life but present a picture of ancient times and nearly forgotten roots more imagined than real: rather like a dead tree which remains rooted for decades without bearing foliage or fruit.

Nevertheless, one or two centuries ago, these practices were still real and artistic expression played an integral part in various rituals and ceremonies. To give an example: the *Roitschagadda* who ran down the snowy fields and the dark streets of the village in the depths of winter: they were noisy, grunting, howling two-legged ogres who appeared from the dead, from the depths of the earth during the longest nights of the year. These creatures were dressed in sheepskins, had monstrous faces, with deformed and grimacing features. If one was not careful, they sometimes took children away. There was also the *Feuilly*, a creature made from young branches and grass, who came to dance in order to summon up spring and who led the whole village in a merry communal dance. So until the time of the industrial revolution, we could say that the area that would later become 'art therapy' was inhabited essentially by local group practices . . .

The social, political and philosophical changes in the nineteenth century meant that the individual took a more prominent place as opposed to the group. Towards the end of this century, the art work of 'mad' people and children attracted attention from those involved with them, and the vigour and originality of some of their products seemed to reflect the process of the dynamic towards individualism. New social groups appeared which had fallen foul of the industrial revolution: adolescents in crisis, abandoned children, unemployed, those who had fled the countryside to become new town dwellers, poor people attracted by the promise of wealth. The development of scientific thought led doctors to consider some of the spontaneous products of mentally ill people as having a function in their treatment and management of their daily lives.

These comments remind me of a similar situation in Bulgaria and the former Yugoslavia, and indeed throughout the Balkans until fairly recently, where whole communities participated in traditional practices, accompanied by specific costumes, dances and music, such as celebrations for New Year, rituals involving driving out devils, or welcoming spring. These practices have also gone into 'folklore', now performed in concert halls or presented to tourists in the major resorts. The same must apply to most European countries, where, as a result of industrialization and urban life, opportunities to engage in these deep-rooted creative activities are disappearing. These traditions tend to get resurrected in tourist resorts where their picturesque quality is often appreciated, but unfortunately gets 'sweetened up' and bears little relation to the original. Communal endeavours can get sidetracked into popular, money-making schemes, such as the so-called 'naive art' movement in the former Yugoslavia, which tended to sentimentalize the past 'village life'. Thus whole areas of communal artistic endeavour have been removed and perhaps with them an important integrative element, which has not been replaced as yet.

Note

1 Further discussion about the Society and the *Centre d'Etude de l'Expression* can be found in Rodriguez and Troll's *L'art therapie* (1995) along with details of available training programmes in France, and many elaborations of terms used in art therapy in France and elsewhere. See also reference list for details of the books in the French language.

The International Society has representation in Spain and Portugal, countries where there is as yet little interest in art therapy, despite attempts by a few British and French trained art therapists to involve universities in Catalonia in training. Indeed participants at a psychiatric conference held in Madrid in August 1996 discussed 'art therapy' when in fact what was meant was the 'psychopathology of art' (see Waller 1996).

Part III

Training and development

7

Training

The sociologists Ben-David and Collins suggest that the growth of new ideas occurs: 'where and when persons become interested in the new idea, not only as intellectual content but also as a potential means of establishing a new intellectual identity and a new occupational role (1966: 452). In the case of art therapy, the need for a change of role and function of institutions of higher education at the beginning of the 1970s in the UK coincided with the beginning of moves by the founder members of the British Association of Art Therapists (BAAT) to find an academic base for art therapy, preferably within a university, as part of their push towards professionalism. There were limited career options for art graduates. Not many could make a living practising their art, and so sought alternative occupations. Teaching did not appeal to many, nor did more commercially-based occupations, so art therapy offered a chance to retain artistic identity while doing work of a socially useful nature, often on a one-to-one or small group basis (see Waller 1991).

The United Kingdom

The first training scheme within the state education system in the UK was in fact an option within the Art Teachers' Diploma at the School of Art Education in Birmingham, started by Michael

Edwards in 1969. This was closely followed by a one-year Certificate in Remedial Art at the then St Albans School of Art, now Hertfordshire College of Art and Design. This college was keen to develop vocational training, and, being in the centre of a large number of hospitals for psychiatric and mentally handicapped patients, saw art therapy as a logical diversification. The course admitted students with paramedical and nursing qualifications as well as art degrees. The Certificate became a Diploma in Art Therapy that received validation by the then public sector validating body, the Council for National Academic Awards, in 1977. A further training in the form of another option within the art teacher education department of the University of London Goldsmiths College was started by the author in 1974. I was then part-time art therapist at the Paddington Centre for Psychotherapy, recently graduated from the Royal College of Art following a period of research into the practice of art therapy. This option also developed into a Diploma in Art Therapy, and a new Art Therapy Unit was formed.

The fact that three institutions of higher education sponsored art therapy training in these forms lent weight to BAAT's campaigns to gain a career and salary structure for art therapy, first within the adult education provision and later in the health service. Art therapists' professional aspirations were also boosted by the growing number of posts that had been established in the latter, although with very poor salaries and conditions of service. Art therapy only 'officially' became a subject of study within the university system in Britain in 1989, with the approval of a Master's Degree in the subject at the University of London, although it had already existed as a subject of academic study at the then Hertfordshire College of Art and the School of Art Education at Birmingham Polytechnic.

I found it useful to study Ivor Goodson's paper, 'Becoming an academic subject: patterns of explanation and evolution' (1981) when considering the development of art therapy training in the UK and elsewhere. The aspect of this article that seems most relevant to art therapy is that dealing with the 'infiltration' of a subject into the education system. Layton (1975) described this process in detail, summarized by Goodson as in the first stage, the 'callow intruder' stakes a place in the timetable, justifying its presence on the grounds of pertinence and utility. Students are attracted to the subject because of its bearing on matters of concern to them. The teachers are rarely trained specialists but bring the 'missionary enthusiasm' of pioneers to their task. In the second stage, a tradition of scholarly work emerges, along with a corps of trained specialists from which teachers may be recruited. Students are still attracted to the study, but increasingly because of its academic status, as much by its relevance to their own problems and concerns. The discipline's own internal logic becomes increasingly influential on the selection and organization of subject matter. Finally, the teachers constitute a professional body with established rules and values. The selection of subject matter is determined now mainly by the judgements and practices of the specialist scholars who lead the field in teaching and research; 'students are initiated into a tradition, their attitudes approaching passivity and resignation, a prelude to disenchantment' (Layton 1975 in Goodson: 167).

Art therapy training in the UK has certainly followed this pattern, although I am not sure that the stage of disenchantment has been reached yet, if applications to courses are any guide. Certainly art therapy struggles with bodies like the UK Higher Education Funding Council, which has a four-year cycle of research assessment. So far this body has failed to address the specific needs of an emerging discipline, which cannot possibly meet the criteria that are set by older, large and well established ones (such as psychology, sociology, medicine). It is both an academic and a vocational subject, so that course content and professional practice are intimately linked. There are also many problems about teaching courses in which the personality of the student is a central feature, which have a high 'experiential' component and in which the ability to apply this to fieldwork is continually assessed.

In the UK art therapy training recognized by BAAT is entirely based in the university system (and there are now five programmes, including one in Scotland which is developing its own Scottish flavour and maintains links with the Scottish branch of SIPE). Nevertheless, they rest uneasily there, trying to compete for funds in national research exercises and with larger departments in their own institutions, and facing the always-present problem of location – they do not fit easily into art and design, nor medicine, nor psychology but are 'too small' to exist as departments in their own right. For the ever-more-bureaucratic and compartmentalizing system of higher education, they represent untidiness. Even when they recruit well (as all the UK courses do) and the staff work flat out to keep high standards, do research, teach and do clinical work to exhaustion point, they seem never to be acknowledged as an integral part of the institution. Nevertheless, the staff and students would seem to maintain a high morale and have not yet reached the stage of 'disillusion' (Layton 1975). However difficult to maintain, training is crucial to the development of a profession and one of the criteria to be fulfilled in becoming a state registered profession is that of a training and body of knowledge that can be examined (in the terms of formal university examinations).

The question of who practises or perhaps rather, who should practise, art therapy is a question that has emerged very often during my research. I posed this question in Chapter 4 when discussing the European Directive on the Free Movement of Professionals (pp. 56–60). It is a fundamental issue because the sets of values and assumptions that the entrants bring to training with them and how these get integrated with that training will greatly influence the future development of the profession. Here the concept of 'role-hybridization' put forward by Ben-David and Collins needs to be addressed. They suggest that role-hybridization accounts in part for the emergence of a new professional role, in that the individual moves from one role to another, such as from one profession or academic field to another, and is placed in a position of role-conflict. The conflict can be solved by giving up attitudes and behaviours appropriate to the old role and adopting those of the new, hence giving up identification with the old group. But if the individual does not want to give up this identification, he or she might attempt to solve the conflict by innovating – that is, by fitting the methods and techniques of the old role to the materials of the new one, in order to create a new role (1966: 459). Clashes of interest may emerge when seemingly different orientations of training are proposed, with entrants from very different backgrounds: for example, art graduates and nurses or doctors. It is asking a lot of a training to enable entrants from such strikingly different groups to take on the identity of an art therapist at the end. As we shall see, many do not and use the art therapy training as an adjunctive one.

In Britain, as in the USA, art therapy's roots have been in art education, art practice and developmental psychology. Entrants to training have been over 90 per cent art graduates, bringing with them a particular set of abilities and assumptions. Professional art therapists have a strong identification with the role of artist as well as therapist and they are very protective of this identity, as the debate over the title of the profession has shown. Experience of working in various European countries, and attendance at European meetings, has demonstrated clearly that there is liable to be a very big difference in practice if, as seems to be the case in most other European countries, entrants to training are primarily medically or paramedically trained (see Waller 1983; 1984; 1992a; 1992b; Waller and Gheorghieva 1990) and they acquire the art practice element of art therapy through participation in art workshops on the course, rather than through an immersion in a four-year degree in art or design.

The socialization of art students takes a very different course from that of medical or nursing students. Attitudes towards concepts such as 'mental health' or 'treatment' are liable to vary. I have already suggested that there may be a tendency for health professionals to see art therapy as a set of techniques to be added on to the primary professional role whereas for art graduates, art therapy is the profession in which they can maintain their identity as artists while absorbing elements of other disciplines and synthesizing these with their art base.

In this respect, art therapists with a visual arts background are very similar to art teachers in their career patterns. One of the very few pieces of research carried out on art teachers was by Carey Bennet, at the time (1983) preparing for a DPhil at the University of Oxford and herself trained as an art teacher. Her study revealed that art teachers were determined to retain their artist identity. This in part accounted for their reluctance to take on senior posts in schools (such as head-teachers) and for their high morale in the case of poor promotion prospects. It would be interesting to see if a similar situation prevailed today, following the Thatcher government's introduction of a national curriculum, which seems to have limited the freedom of art teachers to some extent.

An extract from one of the interviews she conducted revealed that art teachers divided themselves into two: the 'art' people, and the 'teacher' people, implying that these people have particular sets of interests, priorities and values that have implications for their careers. Bennet says: 'The idea of "dual identities" is raised – "himself as an artist and self as a career teacher", and the potential conflicts between these two identities and their associated roles is suggested' (1985: 122). For UK art therapists, this may account for reluctance to take on 'management' posts, where one's identity would be further split between artist, art therapist and manager.

For people who do not have the identity as artist when they enter training, their role-hybridization process has to be very different. They would presumably have split identity subsequently between, say, doctor, art therapist and manager/consultant. This would also introduce complex issues of professional hierarchy, as I found when working with trainees in Bulgaria. In most cases, it was the art therapist identity that took second place or was even demolished through the demands of the initial role – for instance, one trainee found that his chief always had a reason to call him away from his art therapy sessions (which had been timetabled) for a meeting or other apparently urgent reason. Hence the patient suffered, the trainee got frustrated and art therapy did not (understandably) succeed (Waller 1995: 232). Intervention from a higher level in the shape of the project director, a senior psychiatrist and professor, helped the situation somewhat, but there remained the problem of role change. We shall see later, in Vera Vasarhelyi's description of her work in Hungary, that she had to deal with a similar problem.

It was essential for the training to be supported by persons in high ranking positions in order to 'give permission' for art therapy to be taken seriously. Experience shows in the UK that even where an art therapist's identity is firmly held, they may give up art therapy in the face of pressure from colleagues to be like everyone else – social workers, nurses and so on. This usually happens when someone works in isolation, and the role conflict becomes too heavy. In the case of some Goldsmiths trainees, who are nurses *and* artists, they often get pressurized into taking on a nurse role when on placement, as if that is really more useful or important. Being an outsider in a group can be a challenge and very painful. The role of artist in most societies has tended to be that of an outsider or subversive, so it is not surprising if art therapists carry some of that role. Gilroy's (1992) work on art therapists and their art is important in that it looks at a study of occupational choice from the origins of an interest in art to occasionally being able to paint.

It is my view that this question of who should enter art therapy training is fundamentally important and usually not given enough attention. There are likely to be big differences in personality and outlook between those who choose to do a four year degree course in art and design and those who enter nursing or medicine. If there are not when they enter that training then there surely will be once they come out.

In 1985 in the UK, the Training and Education Committee of the British Association of Art Therapists (BAAT) was charged with the task of redefining the core course requirements for training that had been devised in the late 1970s, before art therapy was recognized by the National Health Service. The committee had previously consisted of representatives from all the three existing training programmes and of practising art therapists. The same composition applied to the 1985 working party. The process of redefining the core course took about six years to complete, till the final document was approved by the annual general meeting (AGM) of 1991.

When the Training and Education Committee produced its report and recommendations, they were very different from the previous ones. The committee had established two basic principles: first that the existing one academic year of training was insufficient (the 'callow intruder' had sufficiently established itself to contemplate a longer and more secure place); second, that the basis of the new training should be psychotherapeutic, the principle aim of the training being to enable graduates to undertake practice in which art and the process of making images played a central role in the context of a psychotherapeutic relationship (BAAT 1990: 2, para. 5).

The report maintained that knowledge, understanding and experience of psychotherapeutic relationships was central to the practice of art therapy and of equal importance was the possibility for clients to make personally significant objects or images within the context of a clearly defined relationship with the art therapist.

It followed that the art therapist needed to acquire considerable experience, knowledge and understanding of the nature of psychotherapy in theory and in practice, as well as an in-depth knowledge of symbolic communication, in words, pictures or through the making of objects and the rituals accompanying the act.

Importantly, at the meeting, the membership strengthened the recommendation that personal therapy should be undertaken by all trainees throughout the course by making it mandatory that they should do so. This reflected a situation whereby many art therapy trainees had entered personal therapy of their own accord. It also reflected the growing proximity of art therapy training to that of psychotherapy, rather than art teaching. An important change had occurred in that the *relationship* between art therapist and client had been highlighted, and defined as a *psychotherapeutic* one, implying that it had significance for the process equal to the art work itself, whereas in the past, it was the art work that took priority.

The members of the committee had found themselves in agreement over the structure and content of the training but were unable to concur over the *entry requirements*. Most members felt strongly that entry should normally be limited to art graduates with at least a year's relevant working experience prior to entry to the training, but some wanted to include non-artists in greater numbers than before. This issue is still discussed but there is agreement that the core entry should be from art graduates. At recent AGMs (of art, music and drama therapy) it was agreed to accept an undergraduate degree in arts therapies on the same level as the art degree; that is, as qualifying someone to apply for postgraduate training and thereafter membership of the profession. Developments in higher education have also meant that there are more joint degrees (for example, art and design with communication studies, fine art and art history) from which students apply to become art therapists.

As I have said above, it appears to me to be of central importance that in the UK the philosophical base of the profession is established in the four years of the art degree prior to professional training. This is certainly not the case elsewhere in Europe. It seems as if no one has yet reached Layton's third stage although the UK might be on the way to doing so with state registration having been established in March 1997. Let us now look at training in some countries within Europe (bearing in mind, of course, the European Directive).

Germany[1]

The position in Germany is complex, with many private institutes offering training without, it seems, proper regulation. Karin Dannecker (personal communication) tells us:

> Education in art therapy in Germany is not based on reliable standards yet. Only three art schools at university level offer training: Hochschule der Künste Berlin; Akademie der Künste, München (Munich); Hochschule für Bildende Künste, Dresden. The latter two art academies offer a certificate at the end of the postgraduate studies.
>
> Certificates have no academic value in Germany; for art therapists this means that their payment is not covered by governmental regulations. Institutions interpret this missing degree in the way that they pay their art therapists, not recognizing that the art therapist often has undertaken two university studies before becoming an art therapist. All three art academies constructed their programme as a continuing education for artists and art educators who already have a university degree.
>
> Other academic fields like special education, art education or social pedagogy include art therapy courses as a part of their training: Cologne: Universität zu Köln, Department of Special Education, degree: Diploma in Pedagogy with a focus on art therapy; Münster: Westfälische Wilhelms-Universität, Institute for Pedagogic Learning and Research, degree: art and creative therapeutically expanded pedagogy. There are two anthroposophically oriented schools with degrees on an undergraduate (*Fachhochschule*) level: *Fachhochschule für Kunsttherapie*, Nürtingen; *Fachhochschule für Kunsttherapie und Kunst*, Freie Studienstätte, Ottersberg. A special form of training approved as continuing education by the government but without an academic degree is offered by three institutes: Artaban (Anthroposophic Art Therapy), Berlin; Institute for Humanistic Psychology; Eschweiler; Integrative Therapy,

Europäische Akademie für Psychosoziale Gesundheit und Kreativitätsförderung, Hückeswagen.

In the private training sector there are about 30 private institutes with quite different programmes. Since the programmes of these training institutions are not subject to the stringent regulations and validating processes like universities or *Fachhochschulen* (polytechnics) standards of training vary widely. The courses are expensive (10,000 to 12,000 German marks), students encounter little rigorous training, and the maturity that accompanies graduate work at university level is often not achieved.

The legal situation for all art therapists is open; professional groups from all training levels are working towards establishing appropriate standards for admission and training. What kind of qualification should art therapy candidates have when they want to begin training? This is a very sensitive yet unresolved issue in the movement. Most private training institutes do not ask for an academic degree as an admission requirement. The problem is intensified by the fact that many people not coming from universities have already gone through private training, demanding the same professional acknowledgment as university graduates.The universities argue that the profession would be much further recognized, if every art therapist could prove competence by an academic degree like a diploma.

In 1991, a committee was established by the government Ministry of Health to research every psychotherapeutic field in order to consider legal registration. This committee recommended in a brief note that art therapists must present a much stronger body of research and empirical data in order to achieve recognition. Generally only psychoanalysis and behaviour therapy have access to legal registration. These professions are normally restricted to medical doctors and psychologists. Health insurance companies react accordingly and pay those professionals only.

Nevertheless, despite all the unanswered questions and unresolved problems, many people do find work as art therapists; clinical practice can be done mainly in institutions: psychiatric and psychosomatic hospitals, educational or rehabilitation settings, day treatment centres, nursing homes. Art therapy then is an adjunct to other forms of treatment.

Another detailed account of art therapy training in Germany has been published more recently in the *ECARTE News*, 1997. It reflects many of the points outlined by Karin Dannecker, and draws our attention to the problem of who should practise art therapy and what are the boundaries of the discipline. In the preface to this account, written by art therapy educators, Kossolapow says that there are more training institutions for art therapy than are included in the association of ECARTE. Kossolapow lists these as: a foundation college for art therapy with the emphasis on vocational study and special emphasis on practice (Nürtingen); an art academy with a follow-on study course in art therapy especially for artists or teachers of art (Dresden) and a university study specialization in art and creative therapy within the main course of studies in educational science.[2] Examination of these course descriptions reveal very considerable differences in content and expectations (Kossolapow 1997a: 18).

This newsletter also includes a useful review by Hempen and Kläes of Baukus and Thies's book *Kunsttherapie* (1997). Hempen and Kläes (1997: 40) state:

> As is well known, there has been – up to the present day – no such thing as *the* art therapy. It is still to be assumed that theoretical discussions of the subject matter of art therapy are the result of different practical orientations, based on divergent theories as an ideological–scientific background. This eclectic diversity is a positive thing, considering the fact that the diversity of approaches meets the requirements of a clientele and clearly shows the creative interrelation of theory and practice in its positive turn towards the people concerned. On the other hand it must not be overlooked that the eclectic diversity of methods always implies the danger of confusion and endangers reproducibility.

Even if nowadays the term 'art therapy' for all therapies working with creative instruments (such as music or drama therapy) had become predominant, these approaches do not allow for any conclusions drawn on the underlying theoretical intentions, neither in the field of art, nor concerning the field of therapy. Each time the origins of the terms need to be elaborated.

They point out that Baukus and Thies have identified seven different approaches in Germany (several more than Karin Dannecker found) within which there are further differentiations and reversion to other theoretical bases. However, 'they all share a common intention to increase their academic orientation and consider the field of pure intuition to be outdated' (Hempen and Klaes 1997: 40).

If all these seven approaches have an association attached, then the question of who decides the area of competency of art therapists in Germany, and the limits and boundaries of the profession, will remain exceptionally complex. One can see this as an exciting and rich selection of ideas that avoid the risk of making a rigid doctrine of training, or a very puzzling and sometimes contradictory set of theoretical frameworks. Certainly it will pose an elaborate problem for any national German association to take on.

Switzerland (German cantons)

There are plans to set up a 'Kunstherapie' training programme at a Swiss university, which would offer a three-year full time or five-year part time training. The preferred location would be the Swiss capital, Berne, but Zurich and Lucerne are also contenders. Nina Robinson (1992: 8) comments:

> British readers may well find the Swiss situation strangely paradoxical, and lagging behind in the development of art therapy. That very Swiss trait of caution, combined with the ultra-democratic political system, seems to account at least in part for the present rather chaotic state of art therapy here.

Jacques Stitelmann's contribution in Chapter 3 has already focused on the French speaking cantons.

Finland

Marja von Ronkko, a Finnish student on the postgraduate diploma in art psychotherapy programme at Goldsmiths identified two types of art therapy training in Finland (personal communication); in the 1995 ECARTE prospectus these programmes are described. The introduction to the Finnish section states that the concept of art therapy has traditionally been connected to psychiatric hospitals and in the same way as, for example, France, an early interest in the visual expression of psychiatric patients can be seen in the archives and collections of some hospitals, dating from the start of the twentieth century. The oldest training is that of the University of Art and Design in Helsinki, described as 'psychoanalytic' and as 'one field of application to psychotherapy' (ECARTE 1995: 17). The four year programme of 'visual arts therapy' corresponds to a 'special level' of psychotherapy training. The highest level would be the 'exacting special level' an equivalent of which is hard to assess in the UK and elsewhere, but may be about MA level or above. Entrants must have an art degree of three to four years duration or a suitable alternative, practical work experience, personal ability in art therapy and be in their own therapy. This course seems similar to the UK model. It is the only art therapy training enabling graduates to be registered as psychotherapists and to set up independent practice.

A new training has just been set up in North Karelia Polytechnic, described as 'humanistic and existential' and considers art therapy as a unique therapy with its own language and models. However, on examination of the course information, we find it is entitled 'Degree in Social Studies – Specialization in Art Therapy'. This appears to be an undergraduate level programme and it is not clear what proportion it takes up of the parent degree in social studies. In any case, this programme requires entrants to have the equivalent of British A levels plus proven personal ability for therapeutic work evaluated by interview and 'sufficient artistic ability and orientation evaluated by a portfolio'. It is interesting to note that an MA in music education with a specialization in music therapy takes place at the Sibelius Academy, lasting six years. Music therapy is state-recognized in Finland. It is not clear if there is a relationship between the two programmes listed and if so what it is.

Greece

Greece shares many of the same attitudes towards art as Italy and France, and the development of art therapy has been slow in comparison with, say, individual, group psychotherapy and family therapy. Thanks to the initiative of Nizetta Anagnostopoulou, a Greek art therapist trained in the USA, a centre for arts and psychotherapy has been established in Athens. Originally this housed both drama therapy and art therapy training. Students who train at the centre come from a wide variety of professional backgrounds and commit themselves to three or four part-time years of training. Some parts of the training are also held in Thessaloniki in northern Greece. This programme is developing along the same lines as that of Art Therapy Italiana, mentioned later on, and has a strong relationship with British art therapists and Goldsmiths College. One of the most difficult things to manage is the relationship of other health care professionals towards art therapy, which, by and large, is seen as not very serious. Strenuous efforts by Anagnostopoulou and her colleagues in presenting papers at international conferences in Greece and elsewhere, and in trying to establish research projects to evaluate the effects of art therapy are having an impact, although the lack of any Greek association means that the work falls on the shoulders of a few dedicated people.

The Netherlands

Here the situation is entirely different. The ECARTE directory lists the training programmes in art, drama and music therapy in the Netherlands and the preface states that in the Dutch educational system, one law exists for all the higher educational courses. There is a distinction between universities and the so-called *hogescholen* although both have the same structure and duration of degrees – four years full time of which the first is a 'foundation' year. The universities tend to be more research-based and the *hogescholen* have a greater emphasis on vocational training. All the arts therapy courses are in the *hogescholen* and are financed by the Ministry of Education, Culture and Science. The diplomas are also approved by this ministry. There are five *hogescholen* offering arts therapy programmes and four out of five have courses for two or more art modalities.

The significance of these programmes is that they are open to young students, post-high school, and they do not have a requirement for personal therapy, as do most of the other (postgraduate programmes) mentioned. Although large numbers of students enter the profession, an equally large number drop out. Attempts to deliver a postgraduate diploma programme on similar lines to that in the UK system did not succeed although there are now two Dutch master's degrees in place roughly equating to the British postgraduate diploma.

Italy

Here the situation is very complex with many programmes at different levels and in public and private sector institutions. Mimma della Cagnoletta did some research on the available training and differentiated between training programmes in art therapy (which have stable locations for courses, a broad and/or stable teaching staff, a course of study with a curriculum, a body of courses, a minimum number of hours for internship and supervision), and short courses in art therapy, 'foundation' courses, that run over a short period of time (two, four or six months, or a year) offering mainly practical experience through art therapy modalities.
To the first group belong:

> The ADEG training programme [see also pages 121–3], called the School for Expressive, Non-verbal Psychotherapy, in Turin offers a two-year course for *'educatori, operatori, animatori'* nurses and teachers and a four-year course for a university degree in Psychology or Medicine or Social Studies. Both modes are part-time and cater for students coming from different parts of Italy.
>
> The four-year mode comprises four summer intensive institutes with seminars and four winter intensive institutes with seminars and supervision. For each intensive institute the students have to write papers and a final thesis. The two-year mode comprises only two summer and two winter institutes. Essays and a thesis are requested. Students enrolled in the four-year mode are required to be in personal therapy.

This programme was originally linked with New York University and still has some teachers from NYU (even though the link is no longer official). The teaching staff also includes artists, former students now graduated, psychiatrists, psychologists, an art critic and historian, from the Universities of Turin, Milan and Bologna.

The School of Pedagogical and Artistic Therapy (La Metamorfosi) trains students using the philosophy of Rudolph Steiner. They offer a four-year part-time training. The first year is educational; from the second year the school teaches 450 hours per year of theory and practice including psychopathology, general medicine, Steiner's approach to it, psychology, other approaches to art therapy, watercolour techniques, drawing techniques, clay modelling, other aspects of Steiner's philosophy, Goethe's colour theory, and fairy tale telling.

The school for training '*operatori*' in art therapy, organized by the Centre of Study in Dance and Movement of Florence, began in October 1995.

There are several introductory courses (in Genoa, for instance, and in Milan, organized by a member of the *Comitato Italiano per le Arti Terapie*) which do not lead to any further exploration or training (thus leaving the participants to think they have been trained!). What they essentially provide is personal experience through art therapy modalities. Unfortunately this difference is not clear for either the participants or the leaders, thus giving rise to many misunderstandings and problems.[3]

These examples from various countries demonstrate the difficulty ahead when thinking about the European Directive. There are many different levels and astonishingly varied syllabuses even within the same country, which constitute art therapy training.

Partnerships in training

In considering some of the issues discussed so far, concerning the wide variations in understanding the term art therapy and the deviations in training content and standards, it may be that a useful way forward is to establish partnerships between already existing courses in countries where art therapy is regulated and institutions that now offer similar courses in countries where art therapy is not yet regulated, such as Goldsmiths University of London and Institut pour Perfectionnement (INPER), Switzerland, Art Therapy Italiana and Centro Italiano di Solidarieta (CEIS), Rome; and the United Medical and Dental Schools, London with the University of Szeged, Hungary. Some of these initiatives are described in Vera Vasarhelyi's (Hungary) and Mimma della Cagnoletta's (Italy) contributions. The important thing about the partnership arrangement is that it is not franchising – that is to say, the programmes that develop take into account the specific conditions of the *host* country rather than the offering one. Dialogue between partners could reveal what kinds of issues are likely to be problematic in setting up training, and, importantly, locating a place to practise for the graduates. As I mentioned in the introduction to this book, many of my ideas about training and development of art therapy were tested out during a period of work under the auspices of the World Health Organization at the Medical Academy in Sofia. What had been an informal series of workshops developed into an experimental training programme, which also had a research component (see Waller 1995). Unfortunately, devastating economic difficulties around the late 1980s, together with the upheavals caused throughout eastern Europe, brought a pause in this project, which is on hold in the care of Jhenya and Roumen Gheorghievi, the co-directors of the original project. Very few of the original structures in which the project was based remain, and many personnel have gone abroad or moved to different professions. Nevertheless, for me it was an important and indeed difficult learning experience. As Jhenia Gheorghieva says, art therapy played a part in 'opening a closed system' of psychosocial treatment, which was a rather unexpected outcome of this project (Waller and Gheorghieva 1990).

When I began to work in Bulgaria in 1980, there was already a tradition of art therapy, albeit in the form of art for diagnostic purposes, which had been pioneered by Professor Alexander Marinow, formerly Chief of the Bela Psychiatric Hospital. Marinow wrote and travelled extensively, often under the auspices of the SIPE. We began corresponding back in 1972 and Professor Marinow has remained a champion of art therapy, especially in work with schizophrenic patients, throughout his working life. He had a studio in his hospital in Bela and employed an artist to help patients produce the paintings that he later used with them in friendly 'talking' sessions. As I found, when working in Bulgaria in the early 1980s, the idea of art graduates becoming therapists, or indeed taking on any health-related job was unthinkable – it would not have occurred to anyone to do such a thing. Art graduates expected to work as artists, employed by the state. There was a strict quota of entrants to the various academies and they were trained to expect to practise their profession as members of the artists' union. In Bulgaria they were among the most privileged professionals, occupying some of the best apartments and being able to travel widely. The standard of art produced by students and graduates was technically very high, and, contrary to the views of most western critics, showed plenty of originality. Public commissions were undertaken, which could be prescribed, but on the other hand the rewards were considerable. We might contrast this to the situation of UK fine art graduates, approximately 5 per cent of whom could expect to earn a living practising their art and for whom art therapy makes a very acceptable career. So the participants in the first Bulgarian training programme were 80 per cent psychiatrists with the rest being psychologists and other health professionals. This situation echoes that found by London-based Vera Vasarhelyi in the following account of developing the first visual psychotherapy training in Hungary:

> My own initial ideas of a model, similar to the well-established British one, for collaboration with Hungarian institutions had to be completely reassessed as the professional relationship progressed from an informal to a formal one. The Hungarian tradition of institutions, the traditional role of professions and the particular Hungarian tradition of psychotherapeutic thinking, determined a new model. This encompassed the synthesis of my own British training, a Hungarian way of thinking and the necessity to integrate both into the reality of the fundamental changes in Hungary which were taking place in the late 80s.

I visited Hungary with Professor Cox in November 1990, when we decided to formalize a plan for a postgraduate art psychotherapy course within the context of both Guy's and Szeged Medical Schools, with special emphasis on working with children. This seemed to be an attractive proposition, as child psychiatry in Hungary had a leading role nationwide. There was already a major Tempus programme running with Glasgow and West Germany and a leading Hungarian psychiatrist, Dr Agnes Vetro from Szeged, was in the process of writing the first up-to-date handbook of child psychiatry in eastern Europe. The course content was drawn up and a document jointly formulated, which outlined the aims and objectives of the art psychotherapy course. This paper was submitted to the British Council in Budapest on our way back to Britain. The British Council soon approved the plan under its Academic Link programme and secured the appropriate finances for two academic years. On the basis of the success of the course, the funding was extended for a further year until April 1994. The money was to cover four journeys a year to Hungary by myself, accompanied once a year by one of our consultant child psychiatrists.

Hungarian trainees were to spend time twice yearly on art psychotherapy supervision at the Department of Child and Adolescent Psychiatry in Guy's and St Thomas's Hospitals, London. This provided a further opportunity for them to participate in the training programme of our academic department, including exposure to developmental psychology, child psychiatry and child psychotherapy. In 1993, on the basis of the Hungarian experience, a new course, the child art psychotherapy course, started in the United Medical and Dental School (UMDS) of Guy's and St Thomas's Hospitals, University of London, validated by its Higher Degrees Committee. In the same year also the visual psychotherapy course at the Szent-Gyorgi Medical School received accreditation from UMDS.

It seems to me that the definition of professional identity needs to be organically integrated right from the planning stage into any successful training programme. Considering the history and development of psychoanalysis and psychotherapy in Hungary, it was clear that if the decision was to follow the American and British model – which originated from art education and derived among others from the practice of inspired artists such as Edward Adamson – art therapy would have remained part of occupational therapy for the foreseeable future. The notion that only psychologists and psychiatrists are capable of training and practising as independent therapists is still as strongly held a belief in Hungary today as it was 70 years ago. In order to delineate the philosophy of the Hungarian course properly, two factors had to be considered: first, the development of my own theoretical assumptions based on my clinical practice of art psychotherapy as I experienced it over the last decade in the framework of the medical establishment of a teaching hospital in London; and second, the Hungarian view of the role of the therapist within the institutional hierarchy.

Immediately after my graduation from Goldsmiths College I started to work at the Department of Child and Adolescent Psychiatry at Guy's Hospital. My work was clearly focused on the unconscious processes manifested in images and the therapeutic relationship between myself and my young clients. However, I soon realized that unless I found a consensus with the strong medical–cognitive–behavioural and developmental trends prevailing in the clinic, art psychotherapy was going to be marginalized. 'Doctors have the pill, psychologists the tests, social workers statutory powers. We, of course, all use pictures in our work here and there. What is it all that you, the art psychotherapist, can give us over and above this?' asked one of the senior members of the clinic. I had no choice but to formulate and delineate an identity that could make sense to my colleagues as well as protect the undiluted psychotherapeutic work with images. The need for a definition of my identity and my boundaries, the pressure to reconcile it with an existing structure was also in retrospect a very useful exercise. I realized that the integration of art psychotherapy into the complex system of child psychiatry services had to be a two-way process. I also had to learn to think in other models, to understand my colleagues' formulation of a different, social aspect of the child's problem while I was working with the same child's inner world and unconscious fantasies. It took some time for all of us to learn that all of us were right within our frame of reference. I felt intrigued by models developed and used by psychologists, social workers and psychiatrists, despite my roots in the psychodynamic system of understanding the processes of the human mind. This was the first step in realizing the need to include different modalities in any future specialist training for art psychotherapists wishing to work in a child psychiatry setting. The metamorphosis of my initial assumptions during my 10 years of clinical experience within the multidisciplinary setting was as crucial in determining the nature of the new Hungarian-based course as the understanding of the structure of the institutions in Hungary. This meant that I had to face up to making painful choices between fulfilling the criteria in qualifications set out by the Hungarian psychotherapy training body, or insist on opening up the course to art graduates as well as to psychiatrists and psychologists. Initially I hoped that I would be able to include art graduates with experience in working for the caring professions prior to commencing on the course. However, the fact was that despite attending the same course as the psychiatrists and psychologists, this group of professionals could not become independent practitioners after the course. This meant that art graduates participating on the course would still be able to be employed only on an occupational therapy grade and the level of their therapeutic activity reduced to a little bit of creative activity with the mentally ill.

After careful consideration I came to the conclusion that recognition as a valid form of psychotherapy was more important for the future than the open accessibility of the course.
(Vasarhelyi personal communication)[4]

Another example of a partnership between an existing course and a UK university is that of the postgraduate Diploma in Art Psychotherapy of Art Therapy Italiana (ATI), based in Bologna, and Goldsmiths College. This is a long established training that previously had links with New York University and since 1992 has been validated by Goldsmiths College, University of London. The programme is different from the Goldsmiths postgraduate Diploma in Art Psychotherapy, but meets the stringent requirements for organization of curriculum, teaching standards and quality control, including structure of assessment and examination.

The programme accepts students with a university or university-level degree, after a foundation course of 15 hours and an interview. It is required that students undergo personal psychotherapy by the second year of study.

Mimma della Cagnoletta, one of the directors of ATI writes:

> The course takes place over a period of four years part-time; students are gathered from all over Italy, obliging the structure to be intensive. Seminars and monthly meetings take place in Bologna and Milan, with some foundation courses in Rome as well. During monthly intensive weekends, students have supervision, peer group, art therapy group (eight times a year) and seminars (three or four times a year). The body of courses are taught during the year in these intensive weekends. The teaching staff includes mostly art therapists trained in England, USA and Switzerland, who have long and intense experience in the field and recognized status. Both ATI's founders (currently members of the board of directors) were trained in New York at the Pratt Institute. The foundation courses are now starting to be taught by former students who have completed their training with ATI.
>
> ATI provides liaison and formal agreement with public and private mental health structures, communities, day hospitals and day centres, and schools in order to arrange internships [placements] for students. It has recently opened a centre for art and dance therapy for children near Milan, where students can do their placement with the little patients, starting from their third year. The families of such children are usually incapable of providing economic means to pay for the children's treatment, and they are often unable to understand what is going on. A very high percentage (90 per cent) of cases have given satisfactory results for the family, the school and the psychiatrists. The rest have withdrawn the child before any real modification has occurred.

The process of validation by Goldsmiths took about two years, during which time ATI, while retaining their own structure and entry requirements and methods of teaching, brought the course into line with Goldsmiths' requirements. These were mainly to do with demonstrating a coherent theoretical and clinical base, fair and open means of assessment and examination and a method for monitoring the course. Internal and external examiners were brought in from the UK and Italy and the examinations board was serviced by the academic office of Goldsmiths. The aim of this partnership has been to ensure the rigour of the programme is maintained, and to put ATI in a stronger position to link with other Italian universities. This process has already begun.

In an unpublished letter to the author, Elizabeth Stone-Matho, a lecturer and clinical supervisor at both Turin and Lausanne (INPER) art therapy programmes, provided the following information about another partnership:

> The Associazione per lo Studio del Disagio Giovanile (ADEG) located in Turin and referred to by Cagnoletta [see pages 113–14] offers a four-year, psychoanalytically-oriented training programme in art therapy. ADEG has been offering courses in art therapy since 1983 and a certificate programme since 1985, at which point an official collaboration with New York University, Graduate Art Therapy Programme, was established. In 1983, Raffaella Bortino, a psychotherapist and art therapist specialising in work with drug addicts, founded Il Porto, a residential treatment community. At the same time she founded ADEG with the aim of co-ordinating educational, cultural and community activities.
>
> Prior to these innovations, in the late 1970s and early 1980s, Bortino had spent several years in the United States, collaborating with prominent clinicians in the addictions field and gaining experience working in well-known centres. When *Il Porto* opened, it was the first residential community in Italy to uphold a belief in the value of psychotherapy, and art therapy, in the treatment of drug addiction. Previously, treatment centres tended to be run by priests under the auspices of the church, and were modelled on the 'Daytop' approach prevalent in the United States. This was a very highly structured, somewhat authoritarian model and did not lend itself to incorporating psychodynamic principles. As one of the first two secular treatment centres in Italy, *Il Porto* established a new model or the treatment of addiction in community mental health.
>
> The creation of ADEG permitted the emergence of a dialogue between staff from several different psychological

persuasions and workers in the field of addiction. The inclusion of art therapy was a result of Bortino's personal interest and this had its roots in the workshops on art and relaxation that she and other artists and psychoanalysts had developed in the early 1970s. In 1978 she participated in the 1978 World Congress of the Society for the Psychopathology of Expression (SIPE) in Verona. When she visited the USA between the late 1970s and early 1980s, she met well-known American art therapists, such as Edith Kramer and Laurie Wilson from New York University and gave lectures to students on the 1980–81 art therapy programme there. On return to Turin she organized further art therapy courses, inviting Kramer, Wilson and Elizabeth Stone-Matho to come from the USA to teach. Stone-Matho later moved to Grenoble, France and continued teaching regularly at ADEG.

Following the success of the introductory courses, a three-year professional training programme leading to a Certificate was designed as a collaborative venture between ADEG and New York University. As in the early days of Art Therapy Italiana's programme, staff came regularly from the USA. In 1990, due to changes in NYU's regulations, it was no longer possible for the Certificate to be awarded, so ADEG took over the complete administration of the programme and of granting the Certificate. The programme was expanded to four years to better match Italian state requirements for the practice of psychotherapy and in anticipation of moving towards regulation of art therapy as a profession. Continuing collaboration with NYU has been maintained through visiting tutors who teach the majority of core art therapy courses.

As to the actual programme, it is made up of a two-week summer session and a nine-month winter session for each of the four years. In parallel to the coursework of each winter session is a supervised clinical placement. The programme has a mixture of lectures, seminars and experiential workshops, covering the theory and practice of art therapy with different client groups, psychological processes and group dynamics.

For entry to the course, students are required to have either a degree in psychology, medicine or a related field, a Diploma from an art academy, or be qualified teachers. In addition they need to have had experience of work in a relevant area to the programme (for example, mental health centre). They also have to present a portfolio of art work demonstrating competence in creative expression.

The similarity with Art Therapy Italiana's programme is in content and level, and in origin: namely, the original connexion with American art therapy education and the collaboration with an American university. The difference is that Art Therapy Italiana moved from an American collaboration to an English one. Both centres are engaged in developing their own style, while being open to influences from outside Italy by bringing in visiting staff from the USA, England, France and Germany.

Another Italian-British partnership, also with Goldsmiths College, is that with the Centro Italiano di Solidarieta (CEIS), a coordination centre specializing in the treatment of addiction and engaged in the training of staff worldwide. CEIS began as a community for the rehabilitation of young drug addicts, and has evolved through many stages to its present multidimensional form. I introduced the art therapy training at CEIS in 1986, initially as intensive workshops to give staff some idea of the potential value of art therapy in the treatment of addiction and later as a programme taught in blocks over four years to staff of CEIS. This was meant to provide an additional set of skills to *operatori*, teachers and psychologists at CEIS, but as time went on, the trainees became socialized into art therapists. As a result there is a plan for a discrete art therapy training at CEIS, which would include a substantial element of work with young offenders and drug addicts. Perhaps one of the most important aspects of this programme was that it evolved to meet the needs of the group and that, given the trainees had either very little or no practical art experience, over half the course consisted of art practice, materials workshops and art history. Thus it was a very different programme from that at Goldsmiths, which takes mainly art graduates as trainees. It was in this programme that I became even more aware of the difference between providing an additional set of skills to augment a core profession, and training art therapists. By the end of the course, all the trainees perceived themselves as art therapists, although they were obliged to continue to engage in other work in CEIS.

There is another partnership programme at the Institut pour Perfectionnment (INPER) Lausanne, which had developed from their original Foundation programme for 'animateurs' for which there is no exact translation in professional terms in England. The nearest would be 'hospital artists'. This programme, which lasts for three and a half years, is validated by Goldsmiths College for a postgraduate Diploma in Art Therapy.

None of these collaborative ventures has resulted in a franchized programme. In the case study of art therapy in Ireland in Chapter 2, we saw how important it has been for art therapists in Ireland to create their own training, albeit with input from abroad. The same applies to programmes throughout Europe.

Through the work of ECARTE, and through collaborations with universities, it is certain that other partnerships will occur. For example, some tentative moves have been made, at the time of writing, to form a partnership between a Folksuniversitet in Sweden and Goldsmiths College with the aim of assisting the Swedish Art Therapy Association's attempts to establish the discipline there. In Iceland there are foundation training workshops available through the pioneering work of Sigridur Bjornsdottir who, for many years, has worked with terminally ill children. In Denmark, music therapy is state regulated, but so far no art therapy training has emerged (to my knowledge).

Issues of language in European training partnerships

I have been very conscious in preparing this book that the majority of contributors have translated their papers and the information sent into English, so they have already had to grapple with the problem of expressing culturally-specific concepts into another language. However good one's knowledge of a foreign language may be, for most people it seems challenging and indeed very stressful to discuss one's deepest feelings and emotions in another tongue. Reliance on an interpreter, even a good one, is frustrating in situations where subtlety of meaning, metaphor and symbol predominate, as in art therapy training and practice. Exchange of students and teachers is a very worthwhile idea, but are we to restrict this opportunity to those who speak Dutch, or German, Italian or English, etc., according to where the exchanges are happening? There seem to be few art therapy papers concerning European initiatives which firmly address such a problematic issue. One interesting account is, however, given by a student, Aly Fidom, from Utrecht in the Netherlands who did a practical placement in Italy. She writes:

> Although I prepared myself for the language, my Italian was far from perfect. The more I learned Italian the worse my German and English became, in short it was a chaos in my head. In the first two months it made me a bit clumsy and restless. It forced me to make my point simple and short and I learned to be clear. Sometimes I thought they would think that I was not educated that much. It frustrated me enough not being able to express how I am used to in my own language. And that they did not get to know me completely because some parts did not show because of the language. In my approach to the patients I used the difference in language as an opening in contact. They were very willing to help and laughing about my pronunciation has a lightening effect. In another way the difference in language can hold up an interaction. I gave room to express their anger and frustration about this and I had to accept it. After four months I talked enough Italian and I was more satisfied and I think they were too.
>
> (Fidom and Van der Werf 1997: 73)

A fellow student, Andrea van der Werf, went to Australia and although she grew up using English, she still had many difficulties:

> The difficulties began immediately at my first day, for everyone wanted me to explain the creative arts therapy. And that is not an easy thing to do in Dutch, let alone in English. I had difficulties with talking to patients and other disciplines as well and with writing reports, for this requires typical language used within certain therapies, treatments and within the whole institution. My brain was constantly translating, but some words or expressions cannot be translated that easily or directly.
>
> (Fidom and Van der Werf 1997: 73)

From a paper by della Cagnoletta (1990), in which she describes the development of the art therapy training at Art Therapy Italiana, I understand that when the courses were taught in Italy, in English, mainly by American staff, the percentage of Italian participation was only 35 per cent. Now the courses are taught and examined in Italian, with interpreters provided for foreign guest lecturers. The fact that the course is validated by a British institution, Goldsmiths College, but taught and examined in Italian has presented the College's academic board with an interesting problem of quality control, which it appears to have solved by insisting that the proceedings of the examination board are carried out and minuted in English, and recommending that the external examiner, although Italian, should have a working knowledge of English.

These questions are obviously not specific to art therapy but seem particularly pertinent given that we work with symbol, metaphor, nuances and subtleties of language within the art therapy process. Also, and very importantly, many patients have very poor communication. In the case of people in psychotic states, language could be unintelligible to a native speaker. To a foreigner it might be utterly bewildering. For patients suffering strokes, or from degenerative diseases such as Alzheimer's or other neurological disorders, being faced with a therapist who has a poor command of verbal expression themselves could be the last straw. This raises the question of how far we can rely on the art object and on feelings engendered during the session for deepening our awareness of the patient's world, much in the same way as we would when working with patients who have very little speech. I raise these issues so that the significance of language is not assumed to be slight in a profession that often labels its processes 'non-verbal'.

Conclusion

In this chapter I have drawn attention to some of the issues that are faced by those people already running art therapy training programmes or attempting to establish these within Europe. The introduction by the European Union of directives on the free movement of professionals across the Union (89/48/EC) has already led British art therapists to explore the significance of such a directive on the profession. With the State Registration of Arts Therapists in 1997, the British Federal Arts Therapy Board will become the Competent Authority to operate the Directive. In practice this means scrutinizing applications to join the State Register from EU nationals. Given the very varied levels of training – from short courses, longer foundation programmes and fully-fledged postgraduate Diplomas – and the myriad definitions of art therapy, it is unlikely that many applicants would meet the criteria for the Register. Another issue is that of the core profession from which students enter training: in Britain and in the USA, art therapists are normally art graduates before taking professional training. In many parts of Europe, they may come from a background in psychology, psychiatric nursing, medicine or other paramedical profession and have little or no practical art experience. There may, as a result, be considerable differences in philosophy and treatment approaches to take into account.

Some programmes currently available are mainly theoretical and students do not undertake clinical placement under supervision. Neither are they required to be in personal therapy while training. Others seem to be based on one approach, which I would refer to as the 'Guru approach', and are not exposed to critical analysis of theory and practice.

It seems extremely important, therefore, that an organization such as ECARTE, or a European professional association, such as EABONATA, takes on the task of drawing up a core standard of practice, including subjects to be studied, and a code of ethics, which could be agreed as a criterion to be aimed for. The training institutions have a responsibility to their students and very importantly to the public with whom they will work, to ensure that the highest standards of training and education are provided and that these are subject to rigorous quality assurance.

Notes

1 Details of arts therapy journals in the German language can be obtained from Internationale Gesellschaft für Polyäesthetische Erzeihung, c/o Hochschule für Musik and Darstellende Künst 'Mozarteum', A-5020 Salzburg, Mirabellplatz 1.

2 A useful study of the development of art therapy within the field of special education has been made by Karl-Heinz Menzen (1992).
3 To these programmes described by Mimma della Cagnoletta (pers comm) we can add a new course that has since begun at the *Universita degli studi di Roma 'Tor Vergata'* under the directorship of Professor Nicola Ciani, a psychiatrist. This is described in detail in the Italian art therapy journal *Arti Terapie*, July 1997.
4 Further details of the structure and course content of this programme can be found in Vasarhelyi (1992) together with an article by Szilard (1992) on Hungarian psychiatry.

8
Professional development

In previous chapters we have seen that there is a growing interest in art therapy as a mode of treatment for emotional and psychiatric problems throughout Europe and that, although in some countries, for example in Switzerland, Germany and France, there exists an extensive body of literature and several training programmes, it is only in the UK where art therapy has passed through the stage of being an occupational group to becoming recognized as a profession through state registration. Bearing in mind that graduates of existing and emergent training programmes will wish to find employment in their chosen profession, and given the lack of opportunity to do so throughout Europe at present, there needs to be urgent attention to the question of how these graduates are going to be able to compete with other professionals and find a way to offer their skills to patients. Despite the proliferation of associations and societies for art therapy, very few seem to have taken on the task of setting standards and organizing professional activity, which involves convincing government bodies and employers that their service has something particular to contribute to people in distress, and that such skills may be safely offered. Rather they have preferred the 'learned society' aspect of associating, which may help to disseminate ideas and increase knowledge within an already interested group and by chance to others, but does not help to integrate these skills into a national health or social care programme. I have often heard complaints from trainees that they are making a considerable commitment of time and money in undertaking training but they fear that they will not be able to use their new knowledge subsequently. They accept that they are pioneers and as such will have to be responsible for creating opportunities, but, as was the case in the UK, they need to be backed up by a strong group who will lend support to their efforts. This group would ideally consist of a mix of elders or founders and followers, the graduates who have an interest in pushing forward the professional activity and creating new opportunities (see Waller 1991 for an account of this process in the UK).

In 1991 an initiative was taken by a working party launched under the auspices of the International Art Therapy Association, based in Basel, Switzerland. This is actually a German-speaking, multidisciplinary association of persons having an interest in arts therapies, which has hosted seminars and conferences but played no part in developing training nor involving itself in issues of employment. Some members felt strongly that a Europe-wide professional association was needed to stimulate the recognition of art therapy as a profession. This might mean helping art therapists in countries where it was not regulated (most) to develop strategies for bringing this about. Liaison with government bodies and trade unions would be essential in this process, as British art therapists have discovered.

In Dieppe in 1992, during the conference of the French society for art therapy, a proposal was made by this working group to set up a European Advisory Body of National Art Therapy Associations (EABONATA). At that meeting it was felt that limiting the association to the concerns of visual art therapists would be sensible and manageable. However, at a later meeting in Holland, 1993, the feeling coming strongly from Dutch and French representatives was that it should embrace all the arts therapies. When we examine the definition of the term 'art' in French, we can see why this was their view. As far as the Netherlands is concerned, there is a tradition of 'creative therapy' which is not very similar to British arts therapy, but which brings together art, music, drama, movement and horticulture in initial training and under one umbrella organization. The involvement of art and creativity in the field of psychotherapy added another problem to those cited by Lydia Tischler for child psychotherapists. At a meeting in Athens, June 1994, further work was done but there has been no significant development since, probably due to lack of funding to attend meetings, the few individuals who were involved being heavily committed in other professional activity, and the very real difficulty of understanding or accepting others' terminology. From looking at the examples given by Horgan and Stitelmann of their experiences of establishing associations in Ireland and Switzerland, and from studying the British example, we can see that there is a formidable amount of work which will have to be undertaken by a few people. This will remain so if each group wishes to reinvent the wheel as far as their country is concerned. Nevertheless, there is evidence that some organizations are taking up the challenge. The following are but some examples.

Italy

The oldest association is Art Therapy Italiana (ATI), which is also an institute providing training (see Chapter 7). It was founded in 1982 by Maria Belfiore, Mimma della Cagnoletta and Marilyn La Monica, all American trained, with the goal of promoting and developing art therapy in Italy. In 1984 a four-year training programme in art and dance-movement therapy was initiated, taught in blocks and summer schools. Art Therapy Italiana is based in Bologna, but has encouraged the growth of regional groups in Milan, Rome and Florence, which has become more feasible as students graduate and increasingly identify themselves as art therapists rather than, for example, psychologists using art therapy, and wish to find jobs with a clear art therapy identity. Art Therapy Italiana publishes a newsletter and occasional journals in the Italian language and is keen to develop European collaboration.

The Comitato Italiano per le Arti Terapie was founded in 1993 by several professionals working in the arts therapies. They made a formal presentation of their aims and objectives at the European Art Therapy Educators Conference held in Ferrara in 1995 and publish a journal, *Arti Terapie*, for which they have sought international contributors.

The organization ADEG, founded in 1984, is based in Turin, and like Art Therapy Italiana offers a training programme. ADEG promotes conferences, cultural events and introductory courses in the arts therapies for members of the public.

Mimma della Cagnoletta wrote that representatives of ATI, ADEG and Comitato Italiano per le Arti Terapie were invited by the Department of Psychology of the University of Bologna to meet, in order to establish common standards of practice and of training. They do not share the same philosophy, but are trying to come to some form of compromise. She mentions that one problem to be faced is that apart from ATI and ADEG, nobody wants such a prolonged and intensive training, preferring to stay with a two-year part-time programme. There may be agreement on a basic level of a two-year programme as a minimum requisite for entry to the profession, to be followed by a further two years of advanced and specialized training, which would include clinical supervision as well as theoretical courses.

A complicating factor is that the Italian government legislated in the 1990s that psychotherapy can only be practised by those qualified in psychology or psychiatry, and having a postgraduate qualification in psychotherapy accredited by a university. If art therapy is to be recognized as psychotherapy, then art therapists are squeezed into a tight corner; only a minority of art therapy students can be recognized as psychotherapists by law.

These issues are similar to the ones discussed by Jacques Stitelmann in Chapter 3. It would seem to be a wider option in professional terms to use the British example as a model, given that there is state regulation for arts therapy but not for psychotherapy. The problem seems to be to find a professional group as a comparator, which British art therapists had to do during the late 1970s. They chose art teachers and adult education lecturers, and the Department for Health chose occupational therapists to indicate levels of training and payment that could be anticipated.

By making a comparison with psychotherapists, who could be seen as having a controversial profession, as there are already conflicts over ownership between psychologists, doctors and lay persons (the last particularly in the UK), it may be that European art therapists will find it hard to achieve any form of state recognition at present.

Slovakia

Professional development is not far advanced in Slovakia. The movement of aesthetic and creative therapies is not yet ready to handle all its different forms as autonomous therapies (like, for example, therapies derived from the investigations of the Austrian Alfons Reiter), or as integrated creative therapy (for example, like Polyaesthetic therapy). The main problem of progress within art therapy in Slovakia, however, is a lack of collaboration among therapy educators, teachers, social workers, employees of the public health care system, psychologists, musicians and musicologists, who should all contribute to the successful development of art therapy.

There is no art therapy established in psychiatric or neuropsychiatric hospitals in Slovakia. Officially art therapists do not exist in the Slovakian Republic. Nevertheless there are a few attempts to teach art therapy within special education. For several years the Presov University (especially Klaudia Kosalova and Irena Mednanska) and the Institute of Integrated Music Pedagogics and Polyaesthetic Education at the University for Music and Dramatic Arts 'Mozarteum' in Salzburg have been collaborating on artistic therapies.

Russia

An association of art therapy, formed in 1996 and based in St Petersburg, has sought collaboration with the British Association of Art Therapists. This is an exciting and challenging venture as the association is keen to develop a training on UK lines while being attentive to the specific problems of developing a profession in such a vast and complex area as Russia. The first international conference to be organized by this association and attended by BAAT officers took place in 1998. It seems the association has purchased current British and American literature on art therapy and is arranging for this to be translated.

Sweden

Art and music therapists have been employed in psychiatric hospitals in Sweden since the 1950s on an *ad hoc* basis, similar to the situation in Britain during the 1950s to the 1980s. There are two professional associations: the Swedish Association for Expressive Therapy, based in Goteborg and the Swedish Society of Art Therapy (*Swenska Foreningen for Bildterapi*) based in Stockholm. There are no correspondents listed in the International Networking Group Newsletter for other parts of Scandinavia. Discussions with representatives of the Swedish Association revealed a small number of committed individuals who are keen to collaborate with European initiatives. At the time of writing there were no formally recognized training programmes.

France

Geoff Troll (personal communication) believes that France is probably about 20 years behind Great Britain in relation to the professional art therapy movement. He feels this could be linked to the diversity of approach, but also to the fact that French people tend to be rather individualist, each preferring to fight in their own corner, an attitude that has meant that the art therapist's professional identity has developed very slowly. Most French politicians over the last 20 years seem to be more or less open as to the notion of art in therapy within the health service and within the overall social structure. However, as in many other countries, the financial situation seems to be more and more difficult. As long as the managers of art therapy schools spend their time arguing about which way is best, or worse cutting themselves off from their peers, and the federation of art therapists remain weak, the government can avoid creating new posts within state institutions.

This situation seems to have been aggravated by the Chirac era of austerity since 1995. However, some negotiations have permitted certain highly motivated art therapists to transform other posts within their institutions into art therapist posts, but in general they tend to come from occupational therapy and the psychology field. Of course, this has led to great resistance from these two related professions who go to great efforts to avoid these transformations, meaning that by the government's tactics of division, the art therapists have lost two potential groups of allies who feel their own professions are being threatened.

The problems are difficulty of communication and a lack of centralization of schools of art therapy, and a non-recognized level of professional standards. The main tendency in France is that people who undertake art therapy training do so at a postgraduate level and usually in the context of career development (in-post training) and in consequence, find themselves working within an official status as, for example, a nurse or psychologist, and leading an art therapy workshop perhaps once or twice a week as a secondary activity. Most of these people do not identify themselves mainly as art therapists, but as a nurse or psychologist who occasionally uses art therapy; therefore, most of them are not particularly motivated in a professional movement promoting the specific role of art therapy and its professional identity.

Nevertheless, a French art therapy association was created by practising art therapists who felt the need for co-operation between the different movements in art therapy. In 1988 a group of art therapists from several different schools founded the steering committee of the Federation Française des art-therapeutes (FFAT). The first priority of this association was not to establish a principal philosophy for art therapy, but for the practitioners to try to live with their differences and work on the elaboration of a professional identity and standard. They also wanted to develop communication between art therapy practitioners throughout France, and to establish a national deontological code. This group was a solid militant group of pioneers who intended to promote art therapy throughout France by building a national association which would have a strong mandate for the French and European authorities.

The problem in the organization of a national association in France is that France is geographically large, and the number of art therapists is relatively small. Also, most art therapists work for part of their time as art therapists with the rest of their time in another function. They are also generally committed to all sorts of time and energy-consuming projects concerning their personal artistic career, so it is very difficult to get them together.

The federation is now 10 years old and gently ticking over. It will be interesting to see its evolution over the next decade to see how it copes with its adolescence and aspires to maturity. Perhaps this maturity will come with official recognition of art therapy by the government, an official register, or even the creation of a national diploma to ensure that the level of training and the professional function becomes uniform and respectable. Perhaps also we might look forward to guidelines on professional function, criteria of recruitment and conditions of employment.

Austria

Wolfgang Mastnak (personal communication) describes the legal basis of art therapy in Austria and its incorporation into health care provision:

> In former days there was no legal basis for psychotherapy and psychological practice in Austria. Under these circumstances anybody was able to take on the role of a psychotherapist or a psychologist. This situation opened a door to charlatanism and quackery and impeded scientific psychotherapy.
>
> In 1990 the Austrian Republic enacted two laws defining, managing, and legalizing psychotherapy and psychological practice: Law Gazette no. 360 (1990, *Bundesgesetzblatt* 360, i.e. *Psychologengesetz*) and Law Gazette no. 361 (1990, *Bundesgesetzblatt* 361, i.e. *Psychotheapiegesetz*). In order to control and to organize all affairs concerning psychotherapy in Austria as well as to advise the Federal Chancellor on the interpretation of the law above, the Psychotherapiebeirat, a particular expert committee, was installed at the Austrian Federal Chancellery.
>
> The Psychotherapiebeirat is entitled to license or to reject both psychotherapeutic schools and psychotherapists. Psychotherapeutic treatment as well as psychotherapists have to be authorized for public practice. Licensed psychotherapy in Austria is dominated by psychoanalysis and behavioural therapy. Art therapy (as well as music therapy, dance therapy, drama therapy, and body-orientated therapies) is not licensed. For that matter art therapy must not be practised as a psychotherapeutic intervention with outpatients.
>
> Still there are three possibilities to enable work with arttherapeutic methods:
>
> 1 If a therapist, e.g. a psychoanalyst, a behavioural therapist, or a psychiatrist, is fully licensed, he or she can practise art therapy as a supplementary method.

2 Art therapy is practised under the name of art education, recreation, stress-care, etc. There is no legal prohibition to apply art therapeutic methods, e.g. for artistic or developmental purposes.
3 Neuropsychiatric hospitals, health care centres, institutions for rehabilitation, etc. are able to practise all forms of therapy, which do not violate ethical principles and which follow the results of scientific research. This includes the incorporation of art therapy into complex clinical treatments.

Art therapy in Austria is about to be noticed. Currently law and health insurance practice seems to trust conventional drugs and classic (verbal) therapeutic methods. There is, however a trend to accept art therapy and to integrate art therapy in complex therapeutic systems. Scientific research on art therapy and creative acts, which serve as a therapeutic path, are likely to face a hard but successful future within the Austrian health system.

Germany

Karin Dannecker (personal communication) writes:

Several art therapy associations have been founded in the German speaking area, which all claim to work towards establishing the profession: the International Association for Art, Creativity and Therapy (IAACT), *Deutsche Gesellschaft für Kunsttherapie und Therapy mit kreativen Median* (DGKT), *Deutscher Fachverband für Kunst- und Gestaltungstherapie* (DFKGT), *Deutscher Arbeitskreis für Gestaltungstherapie* (DAGTP), *Berufsverband für Kunst-, Musik- and Tanztherapie-Europäischer Dachverband für künstlerische Therapien*/First European Association of Arts Therapies. The existence of five or more associations in such a young field mirrors a great split in Germany. Every art therapist is aware that we are in a pioneering situation.

All our splits and diverging approaches seem to be handled through moving apart in different associations. This is a rather unhealthy stage of development; we know from therapy that splits in a personality or in a family creates suffering inside and outside, not being able to integrate controversial feelings into the whole being. Inside the art therapy community there seems to be an undue lack of communication among people who share the same passions: the love for art and the love for people. Towards the general public it suggests that we don't know what we are doing and where we are going.

Political and legal action is less effective if we represent ourselves as a movement where one hand does not know what the other is doing, where one leg is running in another direction from the other. Politically active psychotherapists from other fields advise that within the various professional groupings one can discuss and differentiate as intensely as necessary but towards the outside, towards politicians and the public we must represent a convincing group that is able to unite and carry the profession with its multiple aspects and diverse approaches. This insight obviously has been acted upon in the British as well as in the American Art Therapy Association. Our work in Germany can profit by these pioneering endeavours. There is no need to reinvent the wheel of art therapy but to learn from what has been successfully prepared by many others. But, as in every new field, experiences can only be integrated on the basis of each individual culture and history. Art therapy in Germany obviously needs to build on the grounds that are cultivated here. Eventually this will help the professional identity to grow.

Netherlands

Art therapy in the Netherlands comes under a general title of 'creative therapy'. There is a professional association: the Dutch Association for Creative Therapy, based in Utrecht. There are training programmes at undergraduate level, with a diploma acknowledged by the government and enabling graduates to work within the state health care system. However, the profession is not regulated and nor is the title 'creative therapist' protected. Creative therapy seems to be acknowledged as a paramedical profession, although psychologists and researchers in the field of music therapy proposed that it be described as a 'semi-professionalized profession'. Creative therapists achieved this position with some difficulty, following a government proposal in 1989 that creative therapy training should be carried out within a much broader framework of health education. The maintenance of autonomy was achieved as a result of support from large employers' organizations in the field of health care, which opined that separate training programmes in creative therapy were essential to its future development and value as a treatment.

The training centres in the Netherlands have been active within ECARTE and keen to collaborate with UK universities in formulating a credit transfer system to facilitate student and staff exchange. There are, though, some difficulties due to the combined arts therapy training and its undergraduate level in collaboration with UK training centres, although work is underway on developing joint 'master's' modules.

Conclusion

In this chapter we have seen how many countries are attempting the task of forming professional associations. In some places the founders have the aim of bringing together the various strands of art therapy practice and training, whereas elsewhere the aim seems to be to remain separate and even competitive. Countries that have regulated psychotherapy (Italy, Austria and Switzerland) may be able to draw on the experience of their psychotherapist colleagues. In all cases, it will be important to form alliances to assist in the task of setting professional standards. If the British experience is anything to go by – and the fact of State Registration suggests it provides a useful model – then enlisting the support of the medical and psychological professions is essential. There is, we might hope, no need to 'reinvent the wheel' and for art therapists in Europe to feel they are alone. It will, though, be important for those founders of professional associations to develop strategies for the organization of the profession, and this will include taking into account prevailing social, cultural and legal frameworks and, of course, of the interests of other professions who may lay claim to 'ownership' of art therapy.

Part IV

Conclusion

9

Present and future

We can see from the examples and from the discussions in the case studies on Ireland and Switzerland (see Chapters 2 and 3), that many initiatives are afoot to develop art therapy. It is quite rare though for there to be a consensus about the way forward.

The latest European initiative that can be mentioned in this book is a round-table conference concerning the professional development of art therapy which took place during the fifteenth International Congress of Societé Internationale de Psychopathologie de l'expression (SIPE) in Biarritz, October 1997. The inclusion of such a discussion on art therapy was one of several initiatives signifying a wish on behalf of SIPE to collaborate with arts therapists. The facilitators came from France, Germany, Serbia, Israel, and the UK. Over two-thirds of the 250 or so congress participants attended and joined in a lively and often heated debate. It emerged strongly that there was some resistance to the notion of pinning art therapy down and standardizing it. Many people feared that this would destroy the creativity inherent in the discipline. Others, however, pressed for codes of practice and ethics in the interests of public protection. Some felt an alliance with psychotherapy would be logical, others wanted to stay firmly with art and artists. The outcome of this debate, which lasted for two hours and involved many speakers from the audience, was a request for more of the same kinds of debate at future congresses and perhaps even seeking space at the next meeting of the European Association for Psychotherapy.

There is currently polarization between those who see art therapy as an art movement, to be practised by artists either with no training or having art-based training with a minimum of psychological or psychiatric input, and those who see it as another branch of medicine or psychology where the art work becomes a diagnostic tool or an adjunct to psychiatric counselling or psychotherapy. There are many professionals who have undertaken some art therapy training and who are glad to use these skills as part of their primary role (as doctor, nurse, occupational therapist and so on). Some have trained in Britain and the UK, returned to their home country and sought to establish an art therapy practice in a public service or privately. Others have formed associations and training programmes, bringing in teachers from abroad, in particular from the UK and USA.

As we have seen, there are many problems about the actual term art therapy, which can mean so many different things depending on one's perception of art, or therapy, and some question whether these terms can coexist at all. As Karin Dannecker (personal communication) points out, 'experiences can only be integrated on the basis of individual culture and history'. We have the example of Ireland to consider, where despite (or perhaps even because of) bitter conflict between North and South, arts therapists have joined together and are working towards a training that reflects their Irish culture but also takes useful elements from Britain and the USA. In Switzerland, a country of three main languages that has enjoyed a peaceful recent history, there are problems in collaboration because of different languages and because of the structure of the cantons. Nevertheless, the Association of Art Therapists Swiss Romande (ARAET) has attempted to contact other Swiss organizations and to start a debate on standards, training and ethics.

In Hungary there has been a long tradition of interest in art therapy through the SIPE and now a collaborative venture between Szeged University and London. Because the trainees are all members of a core profession (psychiatry or psychology) they are unlikely to need a professional association to push for a career and salary structure. The time may come, however, when these trainees become socialized as art therapists and will wish to change their role and be recognized as such.

There is a similar situation in the UK with regard to group psychotherapy and it is relevant to make a comparison. For many years group psychotherapists were trained in the private sector. Entrants to training came mainly from medicine and psychiatry and returned to these professions after graduating. Sometimes they practised in the health and social services, but more often they ran private groups. Hence group psychotherapy remained on the margins of public health care; groups were usually run by untrained conductors, not taken seriously and regarded as of little value. The theoretical and clinical values of group psychotherapy (in common with other forms of psychotherapy) rarely became integrated into treatment programmes. When a training was offered within a university in a department committed to practice within public services, the position changed. Trainees were accepted from a wide range of professions, and included arts therapists, nurses, social workers, teachers, counsellors, probation and prison officers and clergy. After a rigorous training, which included personal therapy, these students identified themselves strongly as group psychotherapists. Their journey was not easy as they had to undergo 'role-hybridization' (Waller 1991: 52–53, 88). Some chose to incorporate their training into their primary role, but many wanted to have a job as a group psychotherapist first and foremost. Despite the existence of group psychotherapy as a discipline since the early 1940s, there was no professional association. The previous graduates had joined a society that was active in promoting conferences, held seminars and mounted regular professional development programmes but did not involve itself in the kinds of activities outlined by Horgan and Stitelmann in Chapters 2 and 3, which were to do with promotion of a profession, standard setting and so on. Graduates of the university training contacted the other centres and proposed a professional association. There was a positive response and the British Association of Group Psychotherapists came into being, with a Council of Management drawn from staff or graduates of all the current training programmes.

Another example of such a UK development is music therapy. The first organized group was a charitable society, which promoted music therapy through publishing a journal, organizing seminars and concerts and having some input into training programmes. The Association of Professional Music Therapists was formed many years after the Society, with the aim of achieving regulation for music therapists in the National Health Service. This association (Association of Professional Music Therapists, APMT) worked with the British Association of Art Therapists (BAAT) during the 1970s towards achieving a career and salary structure, but there was ambivalence among music therapists about the 'political' nature of this campaign, which involved music therapists joining a trades union. BAAT members, on the other hand, had been used to a combination of 'learned society' and 'trades union' aims and objectives. The structure of the Irish Association, ARAET and the St Petersburg Associations seem to be following the same pattern as BAAT, and there seems to be a move in this direction from the Italian organizations. With the proliferation of training programmes throughout Europe, one can be sure that the graduates will want to be recognized and financially rewarded for their skills, that many of them will wish to be seen as professional art therapists, and that members of the public will wish to have access to a safe, effective service. It will be important for the designers of training to take account of the position of the arts in each country, to draw on traditional art forms where these remain alive and to acknowledge their importance as an integrative force in society.

One way forward, then, is to harness the energy and enthusiasm for the arts therapies, which has been clearly demonstrated through meetings, journals, formation of associations and so on, through progressing the ideas behind EABONATA (Chapter 8 page 130). Another way is by partnerships in training, such as those in Hungary, Switzerland and Italy and the formation of a European Network for Research. It may be that the theoretical base of art therapy is strong in one institution (such as a university) in one country, but that conditions for practice are excellent in a hospital in another country. Hence a well-designed 'outcome' study could be mounted, with a cross-cultural dimension.

As I remarked in the introduction, this book is intended to stimulate debate, not to provide the definitive picture of art therapy theory, training and practice throughout Europe. The moment I finished the final draft of this book it was out of date, because other initiatives emerged and some were in the process of change. It would be tempting to try and incorporate all these changes into every stage of the process of completing this book.

However, if we look at the development of art therapy as a process that will fluctuate according to the sociopolitical context, the prevailing economic models, the conflict of interests among groups and nations, then it becomes possible to work collaboratively and in so doing to learn a great deal about oneself as well as one's European neighbours. I hope that this book will be an element in such a process.

Bibliography

Abraham, G. (1991) Folie et anticreativite. *Psychotherapie*, 4: 189–92.
Adorjani, F. (1985) 'Sociotherapeutic creative camp at Pomaz' [near Budapest, Hungary] 1981–85 (brochure).
Association Francaise de recherches et applications des techniques artistiques en pedagogie et medicine (AFRATAPEM) (1990) 'Les bases de l'enseignement en art-thérapie', Université de Tours, St Cyr sur Loire.
Asvall, J.E. (1993) The implications for health, in C.E.M. Normand and J.P. Vaughan (eds) *Europe Without Frontiers: The Implications for Health*. Chichester: J. Wiley and Sons: 7–18.
Bader, A. (1956) De la production artistique des aliénés, *La Vie Médicale*, December (special issue).
Bader, A. (1961) Petits maîtres de la folie, *Insania pingens*. Basal: Ciba.
Bader, A. (1966) Le cas du peintre Suisse Louis Soutter, *La Vie Médicale*, 1066.
Bader, A. (1972a) Geisteskranker oder Künstler. *Der Fall F. Schröder-Sonnenstern*. Bern: H. Huber.
Bader, A. (1972b) Zugang für Bildernei der Schizophrenen vor und nach Prinzhorn, *Confinia Psychiatrica*, 15: 101–15.
Bader, A. (1975a) Geisteskrankheit, bildnerischer Ausdruck und Kunst, Eine Sammlung von Texten zur Psychopathologie des Schöpferischen. Bern: Huber.
Bader, A. (1975b) Psychopathologie et creativité artistique, *Medicine et Hygiene*, 33: 1605–10.

Bader, A. (1976a) Psychopathologie de l'expression dans les pays de langue germanique: essai d'un bilan, *Annuals Medicals Psychologiques*, 134: 381–400.

Bader, A. (1976b) *Zwischen Wahn und Wirklichkeit* (with Navratil, L.) Lucerne: Bucher.

Bader, A. (1986) These-metaphore-chimère (with Salem, G.) Actes d'un symposium sur la dynamique esthetique dans l'art, la folie et la science. Bern: Peter Lang.

Barthelemey, J.M., Bonnet, G., Carroy, J. et al. (1996) *Art and Madness (Art et Folie): Conferences of the Centre for the Study of Expression 1994–95*. Paris: Clinique des Maladies Mentales et de l'encephale, Centre Hospitalier Sainte-Anne.

Baukus, P. and Thies, J. (eds) (1993) *Current Trends in Art Therapy (Aktuelle Tendenzen in der Kunsttherapie)*. Stuttgart: Gustav Fischer Verlag.

Baukus, P. and Thies, J. (eds) (1997) *Künsttherapie*. Stuttgart: Gustav Fischer.

Becker, H.S. (1971) *Sociological Work: Method and Substance*. Harmondsworth: Penguin.

Belfiore, M. (ed.) (1989) *The Problem of Theory*, Vols I and II. Bologna: Art Therapy Italiana.

Belfiore, M. and Colli, L. (eds) (1992) *Almanacco di un decennio*. Bologna: Art Therapy Italiana.

Ben-David, J. and Collins, R. (1966) Social factors in the origins of a new science: The case of psychology. *American Journal of Sociology Review*, 31(4): 451–65.

Bennet, C. (1985) Art teachers' attitudes towards their careers, in S.J. Ball and I. Goodson (eds) *Teachers' Lives and Careers*. London: Falmer Press: 120–7.

Benson, Lord (1992) Speech in House of Lords Debate concerning the profession of Engineering. *Hansard* 18 July: 1206–8.

Beuys, J. (1993) 'Kunst *ist* ja Therapie' und 'jeder Mensch ist ein Künstler', in H. Petzold (ed.) *Die neuen Kreativitätstherapien*. Paderborn: Junferman Verlag.

British Association of Art Therapists (1990) *Core Course Requirements*. Brighton: BAAT. (Available from 11A Richmond Road, Brighton, BN2 3RL.)

Binswanger, L. (1949) *H. Ibsen und das Problem des Selbstrealisation in der Kunst*. Heidelberg: Lambert Schneider.

Bojar, M. (1993) Europe without frontiers, in C.E.M. Normand and J.P. Vaughan (eds) *Europe without Frontiers: The Implications for Health*. Chichester: Wiley and Sons: 3–6.

Boulangé, L. and Lambert, J.L. (1981) *Les autres. Expressions artistiques chez les handicapés mentaux*. Liège, Belgium: Mardaga.

Boustra, J. (1987) *Expression et psychose*. Paris: ESF.
Boyer, A. (1992) *Manuel d'art-thérapie*. Toulouse: Privat.
Bucher, R. and Strauss, A. (1961) Professions in process. *American Journal of Sociology*, LXVI, January: 325–34.
Burley, P. (1994) European Community Directive 89/94 and the Council for the Professions Supplementary to Medicine, in P. Neale (ed.) *Facing the European Challenge – The Role of the Professions in a Wider Europe*. Department of Continuing Education, University of Leeds: 29–40.
della Cagnoletta, M. (1990) Art therapy in Italy. *Inscape Journal of Art Therapy*, Summer: 23–5.
della Cagnoletta, M. and Belfiore, M. (1991) Arts therapy training in Italy: towards a pedagogic model, in M. Belfiore and L. Colli (eds) *Arts Therapy Education: Our European Future. Conference Proceedings*. Hertfordshire College of Art, St Albans: 51–9.
Campbell, J. (1997) *Attivita artistiche in gruppo*. Trento: Edizioni Erickson.
Carr-Saunders, A.M. and Wilson, P.A. (1933) *The Professions*. Oxford: Clarendon Press (reprinted, London: Frank Cass, 1964).
Cogan, M. (1953) Towards a definition of profession. *Harvard Educational Review*, XXIII, winter: 33–50.
Commission of the European Communities (1989) Council Directive of 21 December 1988 on a general system for the recognition of higher education diplomas awarded on completion of professional education and training of at least three years' duration (89/48/EEC). *Official Journal of the European Commission*, No. L 19/16.
Core Course Requirements for Training in Art Therapy (1992) Brighton: British Association of Art Therapists (BAAT).
Cosgrove, J. and Plant, L. (1994) Meitheal. Paper presented to the Music and Disability Conference, Maynooth.
Coulombe, K. (1995) 'Art Therapy in Ireland. Report for the PG Diploma in Art Psychotherapy', Goldsmiths College, London.
Dachy, M. (1994) *Dada et les dadaismes*. Paris: Gallimard.
Dannecker, K. (1994) *Kunst, Symbol und Seele – Thesen zur Kunsttherapie*. Frankfurt am Main: Peter Lang Verlag.
Daval, J.L. (1988) *Histoire de la peinture abstraite*. Paris: Hazan.
Delacroix, H. (1927) *Psychologie de l'art*. Paris: Alcan.
Denner, A. (1967) *L'expression plastique psychopathologie et rééducation des schizophrènes*. Paris: ESF.
Denner, A. (1980) *Des ateliers therapeutiques d'expression plastique*. Paris: ESF.
Department for Health (1977) *Consultative Document on Art, Music, Drama Therapy*. DHSS PM/82/6: Personnel Memorandum. London: Department of Health and Social Services.

Department of Health (1997) *Arts Therapies: Careers in the National Health Service for Graduates in Art Therapy*. London: Health Service Careers.

Dubuffet, J. (1949) *L'Art Brut Préféré aux Arts Culturels*. Paris: Drouin.

Dunkel, J. and Rech, P. (1993) Zur Entwicklung und inhaltlichen Bestimmung des Begriffes 'Kunsttherapie' und verwandter Begrifflichkeiten, in H. Petzold (ed.) *Die neuen Kreativitätstherapien*. Paderborn: Jungferman Verlag.

ECARTE (1995) *A Directory of European Training Courses 1995–6*. Torquay, Devon: ECARTE.

Ernst, M. (1992) *Catalogue d'Exposition*. Paris: Centre Pompidou.

Evans, J. and Dubowski, J. (1991) Introduction, *arts therapy education: our European future*. Conference Proceedings, 1990. St Albans: Hertfordshire College of Art and Design: 4–5. University of Hertfordshire.

Fidom, A. and Van der Werf, A. (1997) The meaning of an international creative arts therapy experience. *ECARTE News*, 2: 70–9.

Forestier, R. and Chevrollier, J.P. (1982) *Art-thérapie. Des concepts à la pratique*. Vouvray: Jam Cantigas.

Franzke, E. (1983) *Der Mensch und sein Gestaltungserleben*. Bern: Huber Verlag.

Gilroy, A. (1992) 'Art Therapists and their art. A study of occupational choice and career development from the origins of an interest in art to occasionally being able to paint', unpublished DPhil thesis. University of Sussex.

Goodson, I. (1981) Becoming an academic subject: patterns of explanation and evolution. *British Journal of Sociology of Education*, 2(2): 163–79.

Hammer, E. (1958/1980) *The Clinical Application of Children's Drawings*. Springfield, IL: Charles C. Thomas.

Haynal, A. (1987) *Depression et creativité*. Lyon: Cesure.

Haynal, A. (1991) Au sujet de la creativité, *Psychotherapie*, 4: 207–13.

Hempen, W. and Klaes, M. (1997) Review of Baukus and Thies (eds), *Kunsttherapie*, and recent publications (1996–7) on art therapy in Germany. *ECARTE News*, 2: 40–56.

Henny, R. (1982) Du symptôme à la creation chez l'enfant, in N. Nicolaidis and E. Schmidt-Kitsikis (eds) *Creativité et/ou symptome*. Paris: Clancier-Guenaud.

Horgan, D. (1992) Bringing it all back home, *Inscape Journal of Art Therapy*, winter: 2–5.

Jacobi, J. (1969) *Vom Bilderreich der Seele*. Olten: Walter.

Jacobi, J. (1971) Compulsive Symptoms in Pictures from the Unconscious, in I. Jakab (ed.) *Psychiatry and Art*. Basel: Karger.

Janicki, A. (1990) Art therapy. *Arteterapia Journal of the Academy of Music* (Poland), 14–22.

Johnson, T. (1972) *Professions and Power*. London: Macmillan.
Jung, C.G. (1971) The transcendent function, in F.C. Hull (ed.) *Collected Works of C.J. Jung, Vol. 6: Psychological Types*. London: Routledge & Kegan Paul.
Klee, P. (1956) *Das Bildnerische Denken*. Basel: Schwabe.
Klee, P. (1965) *Ecrits sur l'art. Tome 1, La Pensee Creatrice*. Paris: Dessain.
Klein, J.P. (1997) *L'art thérapie*. Paris: Presses Universitaires de France.
Klein, M. (1959) *La Psychanalyse des Enfants*. Paris: Presses Universitaires de France.
Kossolapow, L. (1975) *Musische Erziehung zwischen Kunst und Kreativitat*. Frankfurt am Main: Fischer Athenaum Taschenbucher Verlag.
Kossolapow, L. (1997a) Art therapist training within the scope of ECARTE in Germany. *ECARTE News*, 2: 16–17.
Kossolapow, L. (1997b) Art and creativity at the University of Munster. *ECARTE News*, 2: 26–39.
Kossolapow, L. and Mannzmann, A. (1985) *Kreativitat und Therapien*. Bad Honnef: K.H. Bock.
Kramer, E. (1969) *Art as Therapy with Children*. New York: Schocken Books.
Ladame, C. (1919) Guy de Maupassant. Étude psychologique, *La Revue Romande*, Lausanne.
Ladame, C. (1920) A propos des manifestatations artistiques chez les alienes, *Archives Suisses de neurologie et psychiatrie*, Zurich.
Lafargue, G. (1995) *L'Expression Creatrice*. Paris: Edition Morisset.
Larson, M.S. (1977) *The Rise in Professionalism: A Sociological Analysis*. London: University of California Press.
Layton, D. (1975) Science as general education. *Trends in Education*, No. 25, January. London: HMSO.
Leuteritz, A. (1993) Rezeptive Kunsttherapie, in R. Baukus and J. Thies (eds) *Aktuelle Tendenzen in der Kunsttherapie*. Stuttgart: Gustav Fischer Verlag.
Littlewood, R. and Lipsedge, M. (1982) *Aliens and Alienists. Ethnic Minorities and Psychiatry*. London: Pelican.
Luban-Plozza, B. (1992) Per la terza eta: la créatività e la via maestra. *Bulletin des Medicines Suisses*, 49.
Macdonald, K.M. (1995) *The Sociology of Professions*. London: Sage.
Machover, K. (1949) *Personality Projection of the Human Figure*. Springfield, IL: Charles C. Thomas.
Mastnak, W. (1991a) Kunst und Therapie. Paper given at the Polytechic of Vienna, Austria.
Mastnak, W. (1991b): Prolegomena zum Künstlerischen in der Therapie, in G. Hormann (ed.) *Musik-, Tanz- und Kunsttherapie. Zeitschrift fuer künstlerische Therapien, Vol. 22*. Stuttgart: Thieme.

Mastnak, W. (1992) Musik – Tanz – Bild – Szene. Zur Bedeutung künstlerisch-therapeutischer Ansaetze in Kindergarten, Vor- und Grundschule, in *Heilpaedagogik. Vol. 4.*

Mastnak, W. (1993) Polyaesthetische Erziehung und Tiefenpsychologie, in W. Roscher (ed.) *Sinn und Widerspruch musikalischer Bildung. Beitraege zu 'poiesis' und 'aisthesis' heute.* Munchen: Katzbichler.

Mastnak, W. (1994a) Aesthetishes Handeln – Wahrheit auf 'Abwegen'? in *Behinderte in Familie, Schule und Gesellschaft, Vol. 5.*

Mastnak, W. (1994b) Kunst und Künste, Heil und Heilung. Reflexionen und Standortbestimmungen Polyaesthetischer Therapie im Licht eines Jahrzehnts von Musik-, Tanz- und Kunsttherapie, in G. Hörmann (ed.) *Musik-, Tanz- und Kunsttherapie, Vol. 5.* Stuttgart: Thieme.

Mastnak, W. (with Andrea Rauter) (1994c) Künste, Kulte, Konflikte, Polyaesthetische Integration in London als europaeisches Modell, in W. Roscher (ed.) *Künste und Bildung zwischen Ost und West.* Cologne, Du Mont.

Menzen, K-H. (1990) *Vom Umgang mit Bildern. Wie aesthetische Erfahrung paedagogisch nutzbar wurde.* Köln: Claus Richter Verlag.

Menzen, K-H. (1992) *Kunst Therapie: Zur Geschichte der Therapie mit Bildern.* Frankfurt am Main: Peter Lang.

Meunier, P. (Publié sous le pseudonyme M. Reja) (1907) *L'art chez les fous.* Paris: Mercure de France.

Morgenthaler, W. (1921) *Ein Geisteskranker als Künstler.* Bern: Ernst Bircher Press. Reissued in 1985, Vienna/Berlin: Medusa Verlag.

Morgenthaler, W. (1964) *Adolph Wölfli.* Fascicule No. 2. Paris: Publications de l'art brut.

Mueller-Thalheim, W. (1991) *Kunst-Therapie bei Neurotisch-Depressiven.* München: Arcis Verlag.

Muret, M. (1982) 'L'art thérapie', doctoral thesis. University of Geneva.

Muret, M. (1983) *Les Arts Therapies.* Paris: Retz.

Naumburg, M. (1966) *Dynamically Oriented Art Therapy: Its Principles and Practice,* Chicago, IL: Magnolia Street Publishers.

Navratil, L. (1985) Das Haus der Künstler, in A. Marksteiner and R. Danzinger (eds) *Gugging. Versuch einer Psychiatriereform.* Salzburg: AVM-Verlag.

Neale, P. ed. (1994) *Facing the European Challenge – The Role of the Professions in a Wider Europe: Creating European Professionals, Vol. 1.* Department of Continuing Education, University of Leeds.

Normand, C.E.M. and Vaughan, J.P. (eds) (1993) *Europe without Frontiers: The Implications for Health.* Chichester: J. Wiley and Sons.

O'Faolain, N. (1996) Sadism of religious reflected values of society, *Irish Times,* 4 March.

Orzack, L. (1992) *International Authority and Professions. Jean Monet Chair Papers*. Florence: European Policy Unit at the European University Institute.

O'Toole, F. (1996) Sorrowful mysteries etched into bleeding fingers, *Irish Times*, 1 March.

Oury, J. (ed.) (1989) *Création et schizophrénie*. Paris: Galilée.

Pain, S. and Jarreau, G. (1994) *Sur les traces du sujet. Théorie et technique d'une approche art-thérapeutique*. Neuchâtel, Switzerland: Delachaux et Niestlé.

Paulus, H. (1995) Psychoanalyse und Kreativität. Das Erwachen in der Psychoanalyse, in *Texte: Psychoanalyse. Aesthetik, Kulturkritik. Vol. 2*. Vienna: Passage Verlag.

Peiry, L. (1991a) *Charles Ladame ou le cabinet fou d'un psychiatre*. Lausanne: Collection de l'art brut.

Peiry, L. (1991b) *Hans Steck ou le parti pris de la folie*. Lausanne: Collection de l'art brut.

Petersen, P. (1990) *Ansätze kunsttherapeutischer Forschung*, Berlin: Springer Verlag.

Porret-Forel, J. (1966) *Aloise*. Paris: Publications de l'art brut.

Poulton, K. (1993) Health service work force planning in Europe, in C.E.M. Normand and J.P. Vaughan (eds) *Europe without Frontiers: The Implications for Health*. Chichester: John Wiley and Sons.

Prinzhorn, H. (1922) Bildnerei des Geisteskranken. Berlin: Springer.

Prinzhorn, H. (1984) *Expressions de la folie*. (traduction en français) Paris: Gallimard.

Reiter, A. (1978) Psychopathologie und bildnerischer Ausdruck. Die Etablierung eines neuen Forschungsgebietes. Psychologie III. Materialien. Unpublished paper.

Reiter, A. (1982) Bildnerischer Ausdruck als Mittel zur Selbstfindung. hgf forum. Unpublished paper.

Reiter, A. (1983) Kunsttherapie – eine neue psychotherapeutische Methode? Kunst und Therapie, 3: 11–25.

Reiter, A. (1985) Bildnerischer Ausdruck als methodischer, diagostischer und therapeutischer Zugang zur Depression. Habilitationsschrift. Universitaet Salzburg. Unpublished paper.

Reiter, A. (1994) 'Selbst-aktualisierende' Entwicklungsgestalten in Bildserien, in G. Schottenloher (ed.) *Kunst und Therapie*. München: Kösel.

Robinson, N. (1992) Art therapy in Switzerland, *Inscape Journal of Art Therapy*, winter: 5–8.

Rodriguez, J. et Troll, G. (eds) (1995) *L'art-thérapie – pratiques, techniques et concepts*. Paris: Ellébore.

Rorschach, H. (1913a) *Analyse einer schizophrenen Zeichnung*. Zurich: Zentralblatt Psychoanalyse.

Rorschach, H. (1913b) *Analytische Bemerkungen uber das Gemälde eines Schizophrenens*. Zurich: Zentralblatt Psychoanalyse.
Rorschach, H. (1921) *Psychodiagnostik*. Bern: H. Huber.
Roscher, W. (1976) *Polyaesthetische Erziehung*. Klaenge, Texte, Bilder, Szenen, Cologne: Du Mont.
Rosselet-Christ, C. (1988) *Art Plastique et psychologie*. Fribourg: DelVal.
Rougement, T. (1992) Thérapeutique par l'expression, *Confrontations Psychiatriques*, 34: 225–44.
Schaverien, J. (1991) *The Revealing Image*. London: Routledge.
Schmidt, G. (1961) De l'art des alienes dans ses rapports avec l'art, *Insania Pingens*. Basel: Ciba.
Schottenloher, G. (ed.)(1994) *Kunst und Therapie*. München: Kösel.
Spencer, M. (ed.) (1983) *The Healing Role of the Arts: A European Perspective*. Conference Report. (Available from Hospital Audiences Inc., 200 West 42nd Street, NY 10036) New York: Rockefeller Foundation.
Spira, M. (1985) *Creativité et liberté psychique*. Lyon: Cesura.
Spoerri, Th. (1964) *Die Bilderwelt Adolf Wolflis*. In Psychopathologie und bildnerischer ausdruck, Vol. 5. Basel: Serie Sandoz.
Spoerri, Th. (1972) Identität von Abbildung und Abgebildeten in der Bildnerei der Geisteskranken, in *Ausstellungkatalog*, Dokumenta 5, Vol. 11, pp. 1–18, Cologue.
Starobinski, J. (1984) Introduction à la traduction française du livre de Prinzhorn, in H. Prinzhorn (ed.) *Expressions de la Folie*. Paris: Gallimard.
Steck, H. (1961) La mentalité primitive et la pensée magique chez les schizophrenes, *Insania Pingens*. Basel: Ciba.
Steck, H. (1977) Jules Doudin, *Revue l'Art Brut*, no. 10.
Stern, A. (1966) *Une grammaire de l'art enfantin*. Neuchâtel, Switzerland: Delachauxet Niestlé.
Stitelmann, J. (1987) La fiction-video en milieu psychiatrique: du seisme psychique au jeu du tremblement du terre, *Videos plurielles*: 77–100.
Stitelmann, J. (1995a) Art thérapie, ni art ni thérapie, mais encore, *Bulletin des IUPG*, January: 23–30.
Stitelmann, J. (1995b) Une phase d'abstraction dans le developpment de l'expression d'une patiente psychotique en atelier d'expression, *Bulletin de l'ARAET*, no. 1, January: 12–18.
Szilard, J. (1992) A short history of Hungarian psychiatry and psychotherapy in the light of psychiatric and psychoanalytical developments in 20th century Europe, *Inscape Journal of Art Therapy*, winter: 18–20.
Szulc, W. (1995) Training in the arts therapies in the University of Medical Sciences in Poznan, in H. Smitskamp and Z. Fibert (eds) *ECARTE Third European Arts Therapies Conference*, Vol. I, University of Hertfordshire: 11–13.
Tappolet, U. (1985) La thérapie par les marionnettes et le conte du fee, *Art et Therapie*, no. 16–17: 146–49.

Tappolet, U. (1990) Le Conte, la marionnette, l'art du guerisseur, *Art et Thérapie*, no. 36–7: 82–92.
Thevoz, M. (1975) *L'art brut*. Geneva: Skira.
Thevoz, M. (1978) *Le langage de la rupture*. Paris: Puf.
Thevoz, M. (1979) *Ecrits brut*. Paris: Puf.
Thevoz, M. (1985) *Art, folie, lsd, graffiti etc*. Geneva: L'Aire.
Thevoz, M. (1989) *Detournements d'écriture*. Paris: Minuit.
Thevoz, M. (1993–4) L'art thérapie ou l'avenir d'une illusion, *Ethnologica Helvetica*, 17/18: 429–34.
Tischler, L. (1994) Education and training of child psychotherapists across the community, in P. Neale (ed.) *Facing the European Challenge – The Role of the Professions in a Wider Europe*. Department of Continuing Education, University of Leeds: 118–28.
Toepffer, R. (1953) *Melanges sur les Beaux-Arts*. Geneva: P. Cailler.
Toepffer, R. (1965) *Reflexions et menus propos d'un peintre genevois*. Paris: Hachette.
Tyler, R.W. (1952) Distinctive attributes of education for the professions, *Social Work Journal*, XXIII, April: 52–62.
Ulman, E. (1975) Art therapy: problems of definition, in E. Ulman (ed.) *Art Therapy in Theory and Practice*. New York: Schocken Books.
Van, H. (1991) Psychiatrie et creation, *Psychotherapie*, no. 4: 175–80.
Vasarhelyi, V. (1992) Visual psychotherapy – the Hungarian challenge, *Inscape Journal of Art Therapy*, winter: 21–33.
Volmat, R. (1956) *L'art psychopathologique*. Paris: Presses Universitaire de France.
Waller, D. (1983) Art therapy in Bulgaria, part I, *Inscape Journal of Art Therapy*, April: 12–25.
Waller, D. (1984) Art therapy in Bulgaria, part II, *Inscape Journal of Art Therapy*, October: 15–17.
Waller, D. (1991) *Becoming a Profession: The History of Art Therapy in Britain 1940–1982*. London: Routledge.
Waller, D. (1992a) Different things to different people: art therapy in Britain – its history and current development, *The Arts in Psychotherapy*, 19(2): 87–93.
Waller, D. (1992b) The development of art therapy in Italy: some problems of definition and context in professional training and practice, *Inscape Journal of Art Therapy*, winter: 9–17.
Waller, D. (1994) The development of art therapy in Europe: implications of the European Directive, in P. Neale (ed.) *Creating European Professionals*. Leeds: University of Leeds Press. 41–50.
Waller, D. (1995) The development of art therapy in Bulgaria: infiltrating the system, in A. Gilroy and C. Lee (eds) *Art and Music Therapy and Research*. London: Routledge. 223–40.

Waller, D. (1995) *L'Uso dell'Arte Terapia nel gruppi*. Rome: Fondazione Centro Italiano di Solidarieta di Roma.

Waller, D. (1996) 'From Laing to the Lancet: art therapy's uneasy alliances,' keynote paper at the Inner Eye Conference, Talbot Rice Gallery, Edinburgh, November.

Waller, D. and Gheorghieva, J. (1990) Introducing a new psychosocial intervention to the Bulgarian NHS: the case of art therapy, *Inscape Journal of Art Therapy*, winter: 26–35.

Warren, B. (1997) *Arte terapia in educazione e riabilitazione*. Trento: Edizioni Erickson.

Waters, J. (1996a) Crime and alienation: the fruits of false modernity, *Irish Times*, 20 February.

Waters, J. (1996b) There was solidity behind the squinting windows, *Irish Times*, 5 March.

Wertheim-Cahen, T. (1995) Schools and professionals in the creative arts therapies, mutual interests, in *Conference Proceedings of ECARTE conference, 14–17 September 1994. Vol. 1, The Arts Therapist*. Hatfield: University of Hertfordshire. 29–35.

Winnicott, D. (1965) *The Maturational Process and the Facilitating Environment*. London: Hogarth Press.

Winnicott, D. (1971a) *Therapeutic Consultations in Child Psychiatry*. London: Hogarth Press.

Winnicott, D. (1971b) *Playing and Reality*. London: Tavistock.

Journals

American Journal of Art Therapy, Vermont College, Montpelier, VT 05602.

Art et Thérapie, Institut National d'Expression, de Creation, d'Art et Thérapie, 2 rue des Grouets, 41000 Blois.

Art Therapy. Journal of the American Art Therapy Association (English) 1202 Allanson Road, Mundelein, IL. 60060 USA.

Arti Terapie: Periodico Arte, Danza, Musica, Teatro, Video. Associazione Euoropea per le Arti Terapie, Via Felice Grossi Gondi, 50, 00162, Rome.

Expression et Signe, Psychologie Médicale SPM éditeur, 14 rue Drouot, 75009 Paris.

Imagens da Transformacao (Portuguese) Clinica Pomar, Rua Eng. Adel 62, Casa 2, Tijuca Rio de Janeiro CEP 20260–210, Brazil.

Inscape Journal of Art Therapy (English) British Association of Art Therapists, 11A Richmond Road, Brighton, BN2 3RL, UK.

Journal de l'Association Romande Arts et Thérapies (French), 2 Rue des Vieux-Grenadiers, CH 1205, Geneva.

Journal of Art Therapy (Finnish/English) Finnish Art Therapy Association, Lohitie 19A2, Espoo, Finland 02170.

Kunst und Therapie, Ralf Monitor, Bismarckstrasse, 49, D.5000 Cologne.
Les Ateliers Art Cru, Edition des cahiers, 47120 Monteton.
The Arts in Psychotherapy (English) Elsevier Science Inc. 660 White Plains Road, Tarrytown, NY 10591–5153 USA.
Therapie und Kunst (German) International Association for Art, Creativity and Therapy (IAACT), Rümelinbachweg 20, Basel 4054, Switzerland.
Tijdschrift voor Kreatieve Therapie (Dutch) Journal of the Nederlands Vereniging voor Kreatieve Therapie, Fivelingo 253, Utrecht BN 3524, Netherlands.

Useful contacts

This is not an exhaustive list. The organizations listed all have a European or International membership, and interest in dissemination of information on art therapy.

American Art Therapy Association
1202 Allanson Road, Mundelein, Illinois, 60060, USA.
This association also has provision for associate members, as well as being the body responsible for registering art therapists in the USA.

British Association of Art Therapists
11A Richmond Road, Brighton, BN2 3RL, UK.
BAAT is the professional association for art therapists in the UK. It publishes a Register of qualified art therapists and has a category of associate and international membership. It publishes a journal, *Inscape*, twice a year on subscription.
(It is a voluntary organization and has a charitable wing: The Arts Therapy Trust.)

Centre for the Study of Expression
Clinique des Maladies Mentales et de l'Encephale, Centre Hospitalier Sainte-Anne, 100 Rue de la Sante, 75674 Paris Cedex 14, France.
A long established centre which, from 1997 produces a journal of *Art Therapy* mainly in French but with English and Spanish summaries. The Centre also publishes monographs and papers, hosts regular seminars and supports training programmes in Paris.
It has an outstanding archive of patients' art work dating from the beginning of the twentieth century.

Council for Professions Supplementary to Medicine
Park House, 184 Kennington Park Road, London SE11 4BU, UK.
This is the organization responsible for administering the Act of the Professions Supplementary to Medicine (1960). Until the formation of the Arts Therapists Board (May 1998) it was the Competent Authority for arts therapists for overseeing the European Directives on the free movement of professionals across the Union. This duty is now with the Arts Therapists Board. CPSM is a mine of information on all aspects of health care professions in the UK.

EABONATA – European Association for professional art therapy organizations
Currently has 'no fixed address' but contact can be made via the British Association of Art Therapists, 11A Richmond Road, Brighton BN2 3RL, UK, or the Netherlands Association for the Creative Therapies, Fivelingo 253, 3524 BN Utrecht, Netherlands. Aims to make a link between those art therapy associations within Europe that are attempting to promote the profession on a national level. It is run on a voluntary basis.

ECARTE – European Consortium of Arts Therapy Educators
Sarah Scoble, Secretary, South Devon College, Newton Road, Torquay TQ2 5BY, South Devon, UK.
This organization is designed to promote high standards of professional training across Europe. Membership open to courses in the arts therapies that have approval from public institutions (i.e. universities). Holds regular conferences and workshops throughout Europe, which are also open to trainees and members of the public, and produces a newletter and directory of approved training courses. Publications and conferences are usually in the English language, although parts of conferences may be held in the host country's language (Italian, German, French, for instance).

International Arts Medicine Association
3600 Market Street, Philadelphia, PA 19104, USA.
This is an organization of physicians, creative arts therapists and artists who aim to provide a forum for interdisciplinary communication and action between arts and health professionals. It publishes a journal, which is in English only.

International Association for Art, Creativity and Therapy
G. Waser, Rümelinbachweg 20, 4054, Basel, Switzerland.
This association publishes a newsletter, mainly in German, which gives information about European arts therapy events and hosts seminars and conferences. It is open to all interested persons, and acts as a 'learned society'.

International Networking Group of Art Therapists (est 1989)
Simon Willoughby-Booth, Creative Therapies Centre, Gogarburn Hospital, Glasgow Road, Edinburgh EH12 9BJ, Scotland or Bobbi Stoll (Membership) 8020 Briar Summit Drive, Los Angeles, CA, 90046, USA.
This group, which is run on a voluntary basis, publishes an information newsletter keeping various correspondents in touch. This is a good way to make contact with art therapy associations and individuals throughout the world. Publishes, and updates, addresses of associations and correspondents, and lists of professional journals, recently published art therapy books, conferences and meetings. English language only.

International Society for the Psychopathology of Expression and Art Therapy
Dr Guy Roux, Rue du Marechal Joffre 27, 64000 Pau, France.
One of the oldest societies, which has branches throughout the world. Until the late 1980s this society mainly consisted of doctors and psychiatrists with an interest in the psychopathology of expression. At the Biarritz international congress in 1997, its name was changed by the AGM to include 'and Art Therapy'. SIPE publishes a regular newsletter with details of forthcoming events, revues of books and information about the society's plans. It hosts regular seminars and congresses. Publications are usually in French but some are in English.

A useful publication for references to the history of the psychopathology of expression, art brut and art therapy in Europe is:
Macgregor, J. (1978) The discovery of the art of the insane. Facsimile in two volumes printed in 1983 by University Microfilms International, Ann Arbor, Michigan, USA.
This is Macgregor's PhD thesis, which provides a highly detailed and meticulous account of the development of interest in the art of psychiatric patients and 'outsiders'. It has a vast bibliography, including old and rare items, which extends that given in this book and would be of interest to anyone wishing to follow up these references. The thesis formed the basis for Macgregor's beautifully illustrated book of the same title, published in 1989 by Princetown University Press, USA.

Index

ADEG (School for Expressive Non-Verbal Psychotherapy), 113–14, 121–3, 132
adult psychiatric settings, 26
American Art Therapy Association, 159
Anagnostopoulou, Nizetta, 112
ARAET (Association Romande Arts et Therapies), 43, 144
'art brut' movement, 36, 88, 89
art chez des fous, L', 87–8
'art' definitions, 52–3
art education movement, 54, 78, 103
art graduates, Hungary, 119
art-medicine polarization, 144
'art psychotherapy' title, 49–50
art teacher comparisons, 103–4
art therapie definition, 29–30
art therapists' titles, 51
'art therapy' definitions, 47–56
Art Therapy Italiana (ATI), 120–1, 123, 131, 132
Artistry of the Mentally Ill, 89
Association Romande Arts et Therapies (ARAET), 43, 144
Associazione per lo Studio del Disagio Giovanile *see* ADEG
Asvall, J.E., 2, 4
ATI *see* Art Therapy Italiana
Austria, 54, 82–4, 89, 136–7

BAAT *see* British Association of Art Therapists
Bader, Alfred, 34–6
Bauhaus movement, 78
Baukus, P., 109, 110
Ben-David, J., 99, 102
Bennet, Carey, 103–4
Benson, Lord, 67–8
Bierer, Joshua, 84
Bojar, Martin, 84–5
Bortino, Raffaella, 121
British Association of Art Therapists (BAAT), 3, 70, 77–8, 146, 159
  art psychotherapy debate, 49–50
  redefinition of training requirements, 105–6
Bucher, R., 63–4, 66, 70
Bulgarian project, 3, 104, 116
Burley, Peter, 57–8

CAFE (Creative Activity for Everyone), 12
Cahn, Susie, 19–20, 22
Carr-Saunders, A.M., 64
CEIS (Centro Italiano di Solidarieta), 123–4
Centre for the Study of Expression, Paris, 88, 159

Centre International de documentation sur les expressions plastiques (CIDEP), 88–9
Centro Italiano di Solidarieta (CEIS), 123–4
Cery Hospital workshops, Switzerland, 34, 35
child psychiatry settings, 25–6, 117, 118–19
child psychotherapy profession, 4, 58–60
CIDEP (Centre International de documentation sur les expressions plastiques), 88–9
Cogan, M., 64
Collins, R., 99, 102
Comitato Italiano per le Arti Terapie, 131, 132
conflict model, professional development, 66
Cork Regional Training Centre, 27
Cosgrove, J., 14, 15
Coulombe, K., 10
Council for Professions Supplementary to Medicine (CPSM), 3, 57, 63, 160
counselling settings, 19–20
CPSM *see* Council for Professions Supplementary to Medicine
Crawford College of Art and Design, Ireland, 27
Creative Activity for Everyone (CAFE), 12
'creative therapists', 51, 55, 138–9
Cullen, Daniel, 18
cultural contexts *see* socio-cultural contexts
'culture therapy' concept, 53, 55
Czech Republic, 84–6

Dada movement, 31–3
Dannecker, Karin, 53, 89–92, 107–9, 137–8, 144
Daval, J.L., 32
definitions, 47–56, 144
Delacroix, H., 88
della Cagnoletta, Mimma, 72–3, 92–3, 113–15, 120–1, 126
Denmark, 124
Department of Health, 49

designated authority (DA) role, 57
Deutschsprachige Gesellschaft fur Psychopathologie und Ausdruck (DGPA), 82
diploma course, UK, 100
Directive on the Recognition of Professional Qualifications, 3, 56–61
Discovery of the Art of the Insane, The, 161
'dual identity' problems, 104
Dubuffet, J., 88

EABONATA (European Association for Professional Art Therapy Organizations), 55, 73–4, 130, 160
ECARTE (European Consortium of Art Therapy Educators), 55, 61, 73–4, 160
eclectic approach, 22
educational settings, 18–19
Elias, Norbert, 5
entry requirements to training, 106, 108
Ernst, Max, 32
Europe, concept of, 1–2
'Europe without Frontiers' conference, 2
European Association for Professional Art Therapy Organizations *see* EABONATA
European Consortium of Art Therapy Educators *see* ECARTE
European Directive on the free movement of professionals, 56–61

Fachverband fur gestaltende Psychotherapie und Kunsttherapie (GPK), 37
'Facing the European Challenge' conference, 4
Federal Board of Arts Therapists, 69, 70, 127
Federation Francaise des art-therapeutes (FFAT), 135–6
Ferenczy, Sandor, 80–1
Feuilly, 94
FFAT (Federation Francaise des art-therapeutes), 135–6

Fidom, Aly, 125
financing systems, Switzerland, 38–9
Finland, 52, 111
FORUM, 37
France, 77, 87–9, 130, 134–6
functionalist model of profession, 63, 64

gender issues, 71–2
Germany, 77, 89–92, 107–10, 137–8
Gheorghieva, Jhenia, 116
Goldsmiths College, London, 100, 120–1, 123–4
Goodson, Ivor, 100–1
GPK (Fachverband fur gestaltende Psychotherapie und Kunsttherapie), 37
Greece, training, 112
Gross, Otto, 32
group psychotherapy comparison, 145
Guy's Hospital, London, 117–18

Hardi, Istvan, 89
Hempen, W., 109–10
Hermann, Imre, 81
Hertfordshire, University of, 27
Higher Education Funding Council, UK, 101
Hill, Adrian, 48, 77
hospice settings, 26–7
Hungary, 52, 80–2, 89, 117–20, 144

IADAMT *see* Irish Association of Drama, Art and Music Therapists
Il Porto centre, Turin, 121–2
'individualistic' art therapies, 84
'infiltration' into education system, 100–1
Institute of Integrated Medicine, Turin, 114
International Art Therapy Association, Switzerland, 130
International Arts Medicine Association, 160
International Association for Art Therapy, 160

International Networking Group of Art Therapists, 161
International Society for the Study of the Psychopathology of Expression *see* SIPE
Institut pour Perfectionnment (INPER), Lausanne, 124
Ireland, 5, 9–28, 69, 144
  theoretical influences, 21–7
  training, 27–8, 120–1
  work and development, 10–21
Irish Association of Drama, Art and Music Therapists (IADAMT), 11, 12, 13, 15–16, 27
Italy, 53, 72–3, 125, 126, 131–2
  training, 113–15, 120–4

Jacobi, Jolande, 36
Johnson, T., 64–5, 65–6
Jung, C.G., 31

Katan, Esther Dreyfuss, 37
Kearney, Michael, 26–7
Klaes, M., 109–10
Klein, Jean-Pierre, 37
Klement, Berta, 84
knowledge base, importance of, 69–70
Kosalova, Klaudia, 86
Kossolapow, Line, 61, 109
Kunsttherapie, 54
Kyzour, Milan, 85

Lafargue, Guy, 31
language issues, 29–31, 53–6, 125–7
Larson, M.S., 65
Lausanne, Goldsmiths partnership, 124
Layton, D., 100–1
Lipsedge, M., 76
Littlewood, L., 76
Luban-Plozza, B., 37

Macdonald, K.M., 65, 69, 76–7
Macgregor, J., 161
Maltherapy, 38
Marie, A., 88
Marinow, Alexander, 116
Master's degree courses, UK, 100

Index

Mastnak, Wolfgang, 54, 82–4, 85–6, 136–7
Mater Child and Family Centre, 25
McClearey, Bernadette, 10, 20–1
McClelland, Sheila, 10
McCourt, Eileen, 22
McGonigle, Declan, 16
McMahon, Mary, 18–19
McQuaid, Paul, 25–6
medical roles, 104–5
medicine-art polarization, 144
Meitheal project, 13, 14–15
Meunier, Paul, 32, 87–8
Morgenthaler, W., 31, 32
Mueller-Thalheim, Wolfgang, 82
multidimensional approach, 83–4
Muret, Marc, 37
Murtagh, Carmel, 25–6
music therapy comparison, 145–6
'mutual analysis' method, 80–1
Mutual Supervision Group, Ireland, 13

National Health Service Executive, 48–9, 70
Neale, Pauline, 56, 66–7
Netherlands, 47–8, 112–13, 130, 138–9
NIGAT (Northern Ireland Group of Art Therapists), 11, 12
nursing roles, 104–5

occupational therapy comparisons, 70, 71
OFAS (Office Federal des Assurances Sociales), 38
offenders, working with, 18
Office Federal des Assurances Sociales (OFAS), 38
O'Faolain, N., 25
organizational supports, Switzerland, 40
Orzack, L., 67
O'Toole, Fintan, 24
ownership issues, 70–2, 74–5

palliative care settings, 26–7
partnership arrangements, 115–24, 146
penis envy theory, 81
Plant, Liam, 14, 15, 17–18, 22

Poland, 'art' definitions, 52–3
polyaesthetic education, 83, 84
Poulton, Karin, 3
power, professional, 65–70
Prinzhorn, H., 32, 89
private training sector, Germany, 108
private sector work
 Ireland, 20–1
 Switzerland, 38–9
private training sector, Germany, 108
probation service work, 18
process model of professions, 5, 64
'profession' concepts, 63–5
professional development, 129–39
'professional project' concept, 65, 79
professionals, free movement of, 56–61
professions, process model of, 5
Professions Supplementary to Medicine (PSM) Act, 50, 63, 67, 68
psychoanalytic approach, 80–2, 83, 91–2
Psychotherapiebeirat, 136
'psychotherapy' debate, 50, 51, 106, 132

qualifications, mutual recognition, 3, 56–62

racism issues, 2
regulation issues, 72–5
 state registration, 5, 50–1, 67–9
Reiter, Alfons, 82–3
religious organizations, Ireland, 21
rituals, traditional, 93–5
Robinson, Nina, 37–8, 110
Roitschgadda, 94
role conflicts, 102, 103, 104
role-hybridization, 102–5, 145
Ronkko, Marja von, 111
Rosolato, G., 89
Russia, professional development, 133

School of Pedagogical and Artistic Therapy, Italy, 114
school settings, 18–19

Schwitters, Kurt, 33
self-employment, Ireland, 16–17
sickness insurance system, Switzerland, 38, 39
Simon, Rita, 10, 21–2
SIPE (International Society for the Study of the Psychopathology of Expression), 33, 86–7, 90, 143–4, 161
Slovakia, 86, 133
social security system, Switzerland, 38–9
Sociéte Française de Psychopathologie de l'Expression, 89
socio-cultural contexts, 76–96
 Austria, 82–4
 Czech Republic and Slovakia, 84–6
 France, 86–9
 Germany, 89–92
 Hungary, 80–2
 Ireland, 22–5
 Italy, 92–3
 Switzerland, 93–5
 UK, 77–9
St Thomas's Hospital, London, 117–18
state registration, 5, 50–1, 67–9
Steiner, Rudolph, 114
Steps in Expression project, 13
Stern, Arno, 38
Stone-Matho, Elizabeth, 121–3
Strauss, A., 63–4, 66, 70
Sweden, 124, 133–4
Switzerland, 5, 29–44, 69, 70, 144
 finance, 38–9
 International Art Therapy Association, 130
 language, 29–31
 theoretical influences, 31–8
 traditional rituals, 93–5
 training, 35, 39–42, 110
'symbolism of style' approach, 22
Szulc, Wita, 52–3

Tappolet, Ursula, 37
Tardieu, Andre, 87
teacher of art, comparisons, 103–4
teachers, Switzerland, 40–1
teaching, art therapy in, 18–19
theoretical influences
 Ireland, 21–7
 Switzerland, 31–8, 40
therapie definitions, 30–1
Thevoz, Michel, 36–7
Thies, J., 109, 110
Tischler, Lydia, 58–60
trade union links, 78, 79
traditional rituals, 93–5
training, 69–70, 71–2, 75, 99–128
 Finland, 111
 Germany, 107–10
 Greece, 112
 Hungary, 117–20
 Ireland, 13–14, 27–8
 Italy, 113–15, 120–4
 language, 125–7
 Netherlands, 112–13
 partnerships, 115–24
 Switzerland, 35, 39–42, 110
 UK, 99–107
'traits' approach, 64
Troll, Geoff, 87, 134
Tyler, R.W., 64
Tzara, Tristan, 32–3

UK, 54, 93, 77–9
 Hungarian training partnership, 117–18
 training, 99–107
Ulman, Elinor, 53

Vasarhelyi, Vera, 52, 80–2, 117–20
'visual art therapy' definition, 47
Volmat, R., 88, 89
voluntary agency work, Ireland, 19–20, 25–6

Walsh, Noel, 26
Waters, John, 23
Weber, Max, 65
Werf, Andrea van der, 126
Wertheim, Truss, 51
Wiart, C., 88
Wilson, P.A., 64
Wölfli, Adolf, 90
work opportunities, Ireland, 16–21
workshops, Swiss hospital, 34–5